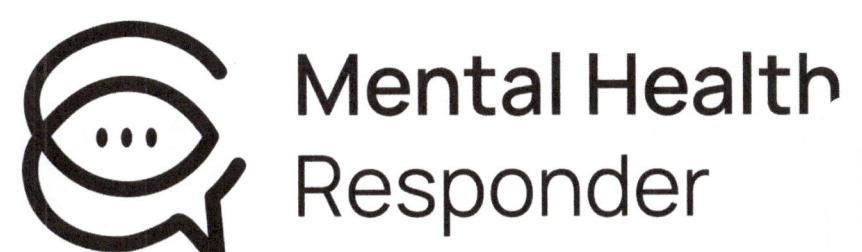 

Thank you for taking the step to improve your understanding of mental health in the workplace. It's about time that we ensure that everyone has the tools and resources that they need to support others but to also support themselves through difficult times.

Mental Health Responder was born out of a mission to make mental health training more accessible, adaptive and relatable. Mental Health Conditions are on the rise, not only is that impacting people's lives but also having a substantial impact on businesses and co-workers.

This course has been created with the end-user at heart. It's been built with what we know is important for you and answers the questions that you want to see. We hope that you taking part in this course starts your journey on a mission to improve mental health and be supportive members of the community for other people.

Mental Health Responder is a programme developed and run by the Be Free Campaign, a mental health charity focussed on prevention and early intervention. Thank you for supporting the Be Free Campaign and our mission to build a mentally healthy world.

Shantanu Kundu

Shantanu Kundu MSc FRSPH
Chief Executive Officer | Be Free Campaign

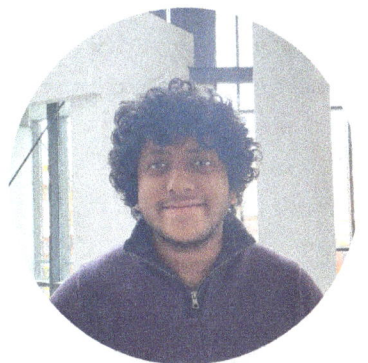 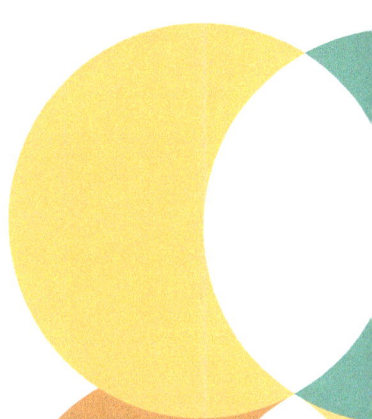

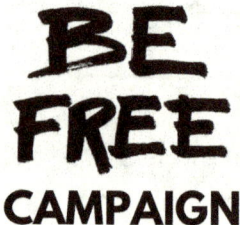

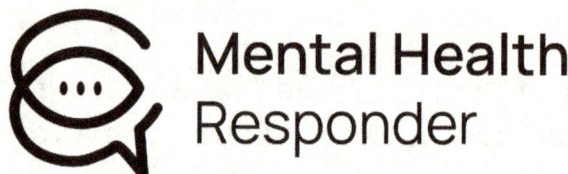

Mental Health
Responder

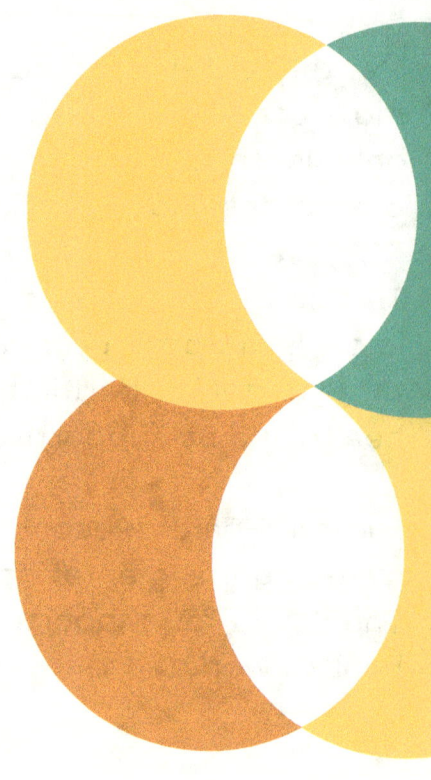

Content within this manual has been adapted from
The Journey - A Be Free Campaign Publication

CONTENTS

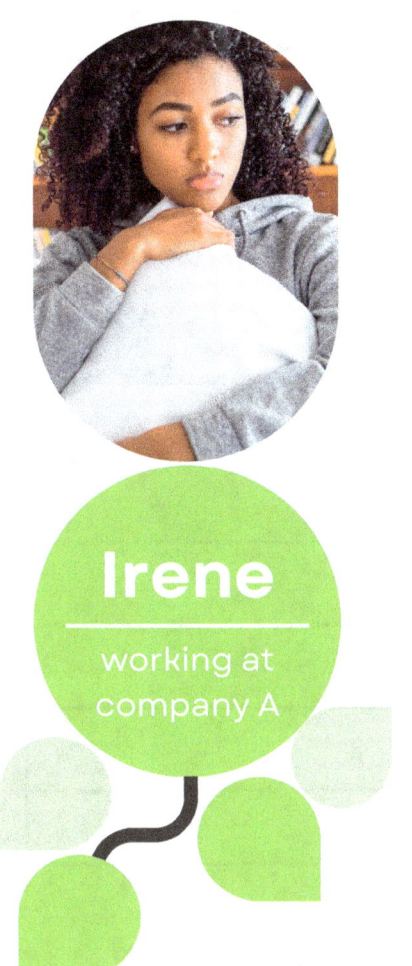

Irene

working at company A

The cycle of Negativity

Irene has been working at company A for three months.

She is beginning to think that her boss doesn't like her and shows preferential treatment to her colleagues.

Irene feels unappreciated and undervalued as a hardworking employee of the company.

Irene starts to put less effort into her work projects. Why bother if they don't value her?

What do you think happens next?
Can you think of ways Irene can break this cycle of negativity?

The Cognitive Triangle

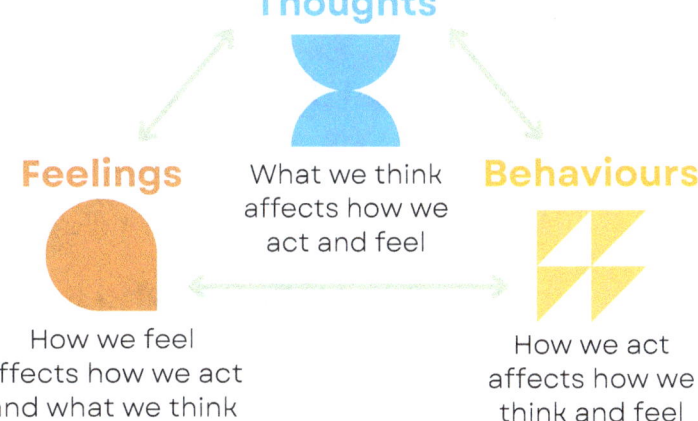

Thoughts
What we think affects how we act and feel

Feelings
How we feel affects how we act and what we think

Behaviours
How we act affects how we think and feel

Coping Mechanisms of Stress in the Workplace

✏️ Chose from the coping strategies below and decide if you think it is an adaptive strategy, or a maladaptive strategy.

COPING STRATEGIES	
Adaptive	Maladaptive

Binge eating, substance use   **Turning to religion**

Regulation one's emotions   **Procrastination**

Behavioural – by taking actions to reduce stress   **Active coping**

Behavioural disengagement, social withdrawal

Perspective - How we think about the stressor

Accommodative - Altering expectations

Self-injury, self-criticism and avoidance   **Venting**

Escaping from the situation physically and mentally

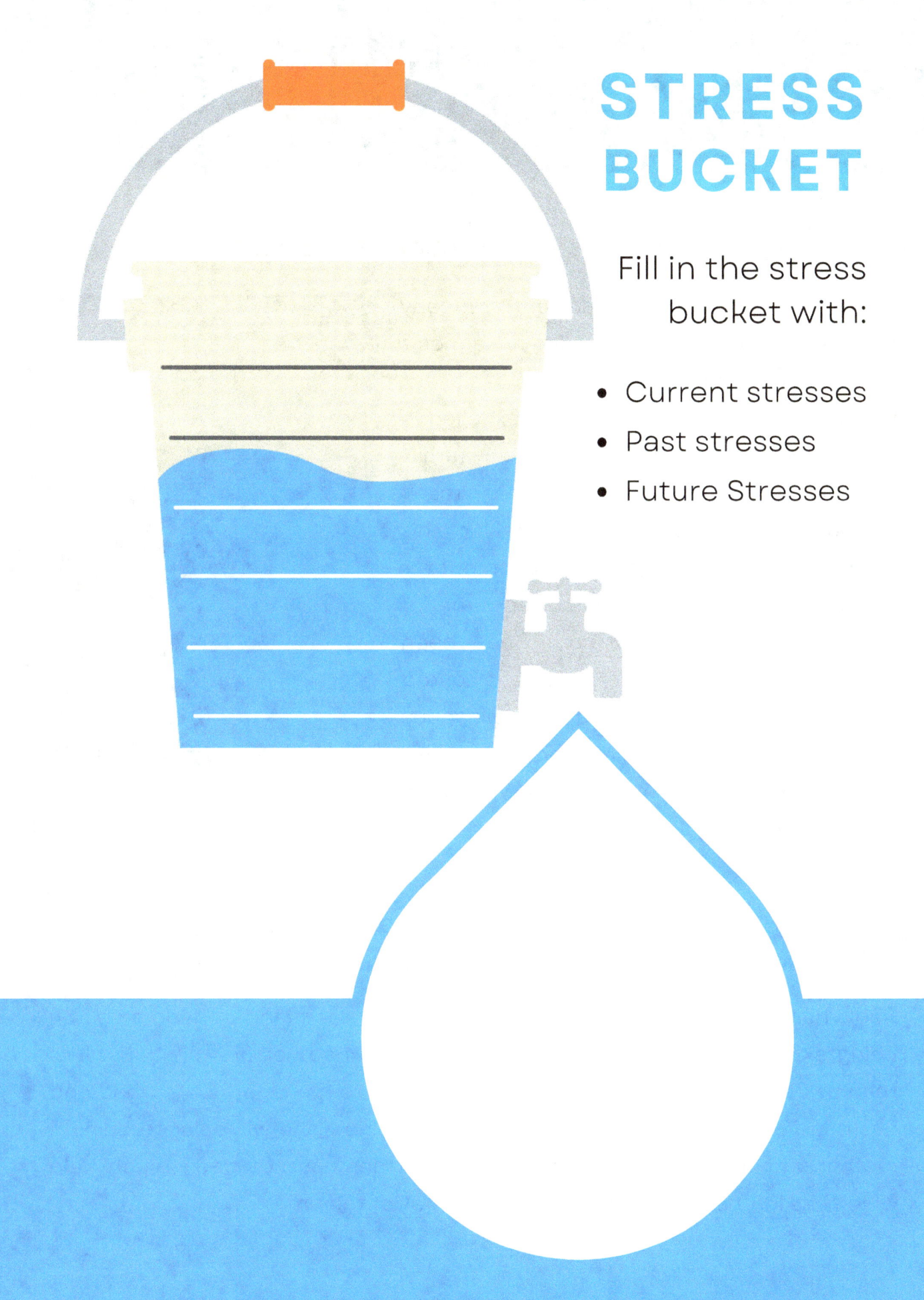

STRESS BUCKET

Fill in the stress bucket with:

- Current stresses
- Past stresses
- Future Stresses

Section 3

Scenario 1 — Diagnosis – poor mental wellbeing

Morgan has worked at his current company for 2 years now. Despite receiving a diagnosis of bipolar disorder 10 years ago, he has never let this hold him back and he has excelled in his job. After a sudden loss in a family member, Morgan has found himself struggling and has stopped taking his medication. Morgan is afraid to reach out for help at work as it is a really important time for the company. Instead, Morgan has been calling in sick almost every day. He is scared to ask for help as he fears his colleagues would not understand. Recently he has started to believe that everyone would be better off without him.

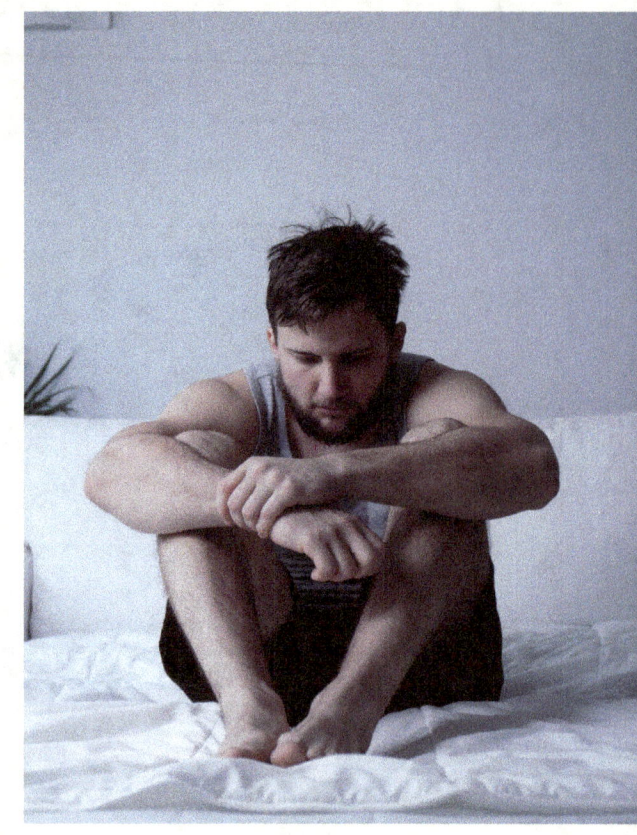

Scenario 2 — No diagnosis – poor mental wellbeing – self stigma stopping her from getting help

Nadia has always been a valuable member of her team and prided herself on being extremely hard-working and driven. Nadia had her first child just less than a year ago, she is finding it extremely hard to manage motherhood and has been crying all of the time. She is worried how she will balance being a mother with her successful career. Her partner has not been much help which has left her feeling angry and moody all of the time.

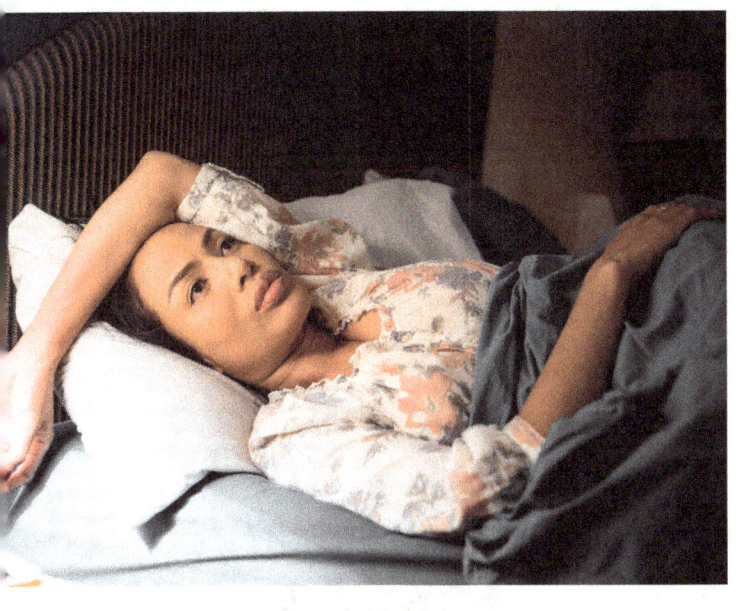

Nadia's sister had suggested she may have post-natal depression and should go to the doctors. But Nadia has refused as she is worried a diagnosis would mean she would appear weak to her co-workers if she has to take any more time off work. Nadia now feels she is failing at all areas in her life and has started to believe she would be better off not living.

Scenario 3   Poor mental wellbeing

Good mental wellbeing

Kai is a recent Law graduate and has just started his first Grad job in a new city. Kai is apprehensive about how he will find his new life as throughout university he struggled with his mental health and did not make many friends. He has been taking antidepressants for the last two years now which have helped but he is worried change will make things worse.

Kai let his new team know that he has struggled with his mental health in the past and they were all very understanding. He has now been in the new job for 6 months; he still takes his antidepressants but is the happiest he has ever felt. He is extremely good at his job and has made some good friends. Kai's team regularly check on him to see how he is doing.

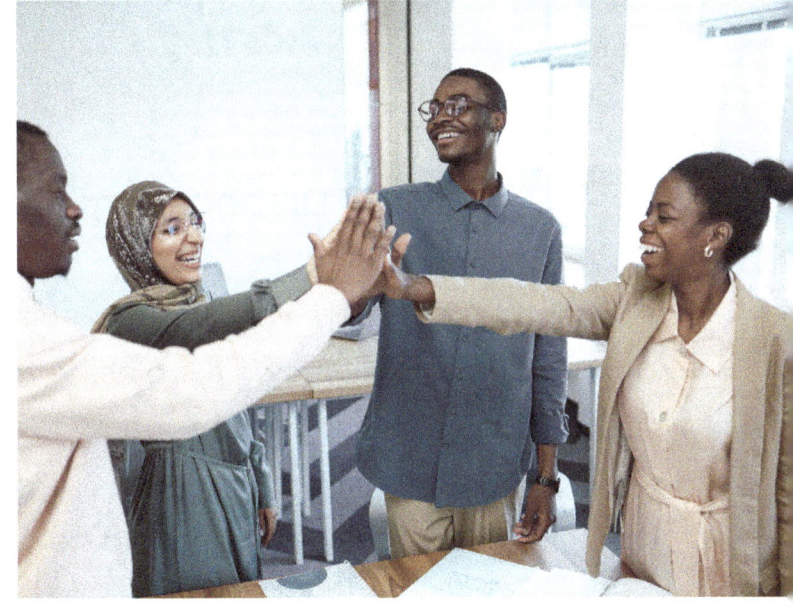

Hospitality

No diagnosis , poor mental health

Emily has been working as a waitress at a restaurant in town for two years now. She has always seemed an easy-going kind of person who is great with customers (particularly the difficult ones). She has always worked well in a team and has been able to keep up with the fast-paced environment. Recently she has become more irritable at work and often becomes tearful when a problem occurs, something she used to be great with dealing with! Emily has been becoming increasingly unhappy, clocking in late for shifts, and yesterday she did not turn up for her shift at all.

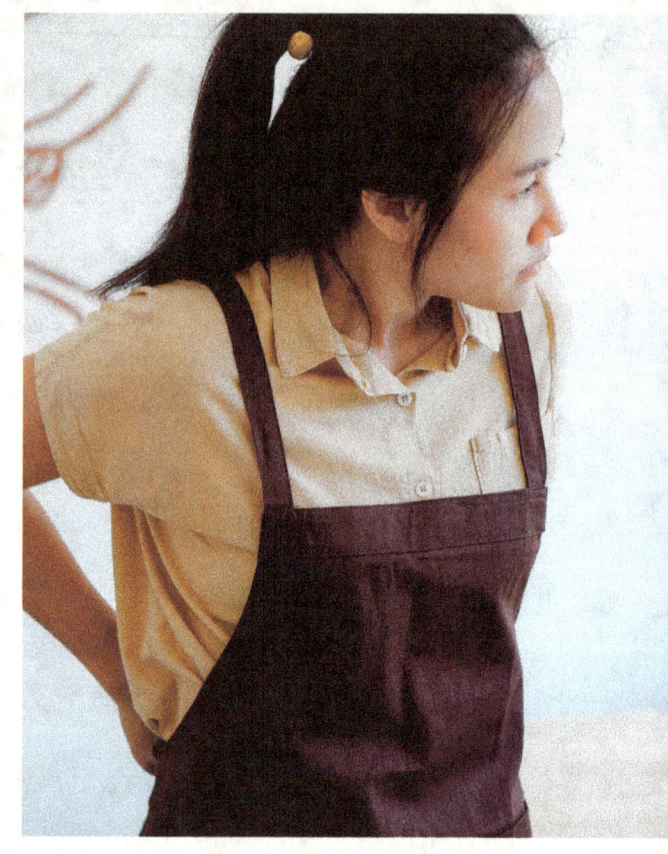

Scenario 2 Diagnosis, maximum mental wellbeing

Joe had struggled with anxiety his whole life and had found it almost impossible to hold down a job as he frequently became overwhelmed and felt as if he was letting his team down. Joe often blamed himself thinking there was something wrong with him. Joe's friends and family prompted him to go to the doctor to see if they could help.

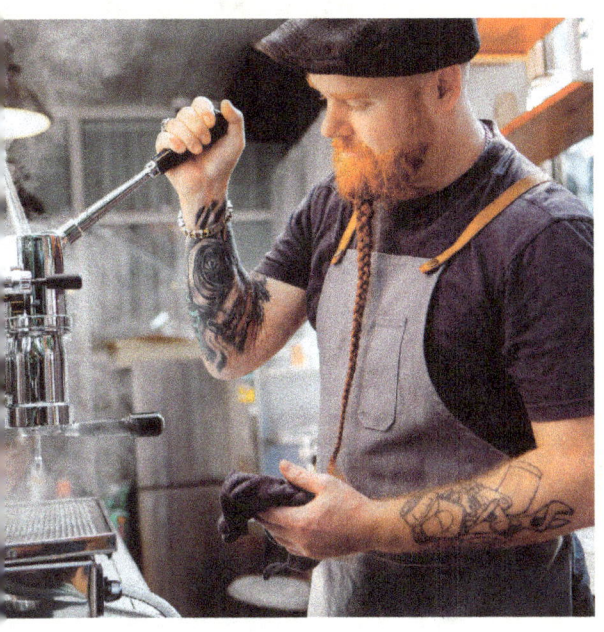

Despite being apprehensive at first, Joe agreed and shortly after was diagnosed with Generalised Anxiety Disorder (GAD). Joe felt extremely validated by his diagnosis and decided to go to therapy and take medication. Since then, everything has changed for Joe. He has just started a new job at the Café by his street and feels greatly appreciated by his teams. Joe still exhibits some symptoms of anxiety from time to time, but his new team are understanding and know how to help him.

Scenario 3 **No diagnosis, variations in mental wellbeing**

Samara has worked at a bar for 8 months now alongside her university degree. She is extremely outgoing, gets on great with the team and always seems happy. Over the past two weeks Samara has not seemed herself. She is often silent on shifts and is making frequent mistakes due to a lack of concentrations. Another member of bar staff, Matilda, notices this difference in Samara and asks her if she is okay as she has been worried about her. Samara admits she has been struggling recently with her university work is feeling overwhelmed. Matilda advises Samara to talk to her shift manager to talk about reducing hours, which Samara does. Matilda continues to check on Samara to see how she is doing throughout the next few weeks. Samara is now back to her usual self, and feels very appreciate to be part of such an understanding workplace.

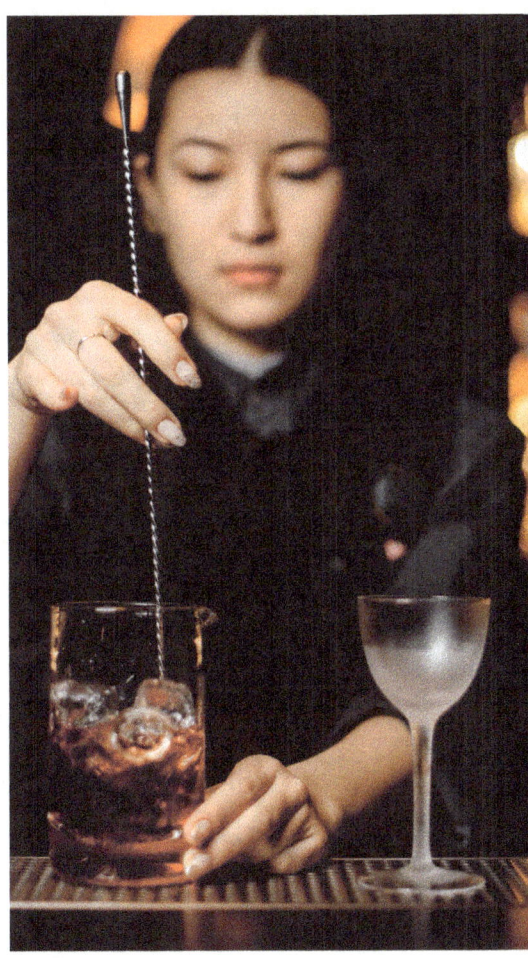

Section 4

What can you remember about the following?

Depression

Anxiety Disorders

Eating Disorders

Serious Mental Illness

Workplace workshop
Activity Planning for Suicide Section

> **Myth**
>
> Asking someone if they are suicidal puts the idea in the head.

False! All evidence shows talking about suicide significantly reduces the risk of it occurring. One of the only ways to know if someone intends on taking their own life us to ask! It can often be a relief for the person to have someone recognise the seriousness of their distress. Asking someone can be an important step in getting help: It can be an opportunity to talk about the situation in an empathetic and non-judgmental manner.

Myth

It is impossible to stop someone intent on suicide.

False! Suicide is never inevitable and can be prevented. Immediate practical help can deflect a person's suicidal intentions in the short-term. Following the ALGEE method will help. It is important to stay with the person, encourage them to talk about how they feel and help them to make a plan moving forward. Always try to seek professional support for help in the long-term.

Myth

There is little warning if a person intends to take their own life.

False! People who are contemplating suicide do often express signs of intent – studies reveal that a suicidal person gives many warning signs. Although these are not always easy to recognise or understand. Signs can be both direct or indirect. If you ever have any concerns, you should discuss these with the person, another trusted person, or a mental health professional. Alertness to these signs could save a life.

Myth

Once someone has attempted suicide before, and survived, they won't try it again.

False! A previous suicide attempt is an important risk factor / predictor for future attempts. It is likely the level of danger will increase with each subsequent attempt. Providing support and guidance when a person has had a suicide attempt can help them see that things can get better.

Myth

Suicidal people are always fully intent on dying.

False! The majority of people who feel suicidal do not actually want to die; rather, they just don't want to live with the life they have at the moment. The distinction between the two is very important and is why talking about it and discussing options for the future is so beneficial.

Myth

All suicidal people are lonely and socially withdrawn

False! Although it is common for people with suicidal intentions to purposefully isolate themselves – suicide does not have a certain 'look'. Not all suicidal people are lonely and not all people who like to be alone are suicidal. Even the most sociable people have their own battles.

Myth

People who talk about suicide won't actually go through with it

False! All conversations about suicide should be taken seriously. Actions can save lives – whenever someone tells you that they are thinking about suicide, it is important that you keep them safe and discuss professional help available to them.

Myth

People who seem to be getting better might still be suicidal.

True! Sadly, someone who may seem to have improved, may be lying to put on a brave face for others, but underneath is still feeling suicidal. It's important to look out for signs such as: being more affectionate than usual, a sudden sense of 'closure' that seems unexplained, or selling things for a 'fresh start'.

Myth

More men die by suicide than women.

True! Statistics show that men are around 3x more likely to die by suicide than women. There are many reasons for why this is true. It may be that men find it harder to talk about their feelings due to societal pressures. It is important to note that whilst men are more likely to die by suicide – women show higher rates of non-fatal suicide attempts and suicidal ideation.

Myth

LGBTQ people are at higher risk of suicide

True! Statistically, those from the LGBTQ+ community are at a higher risk of suicidal thoughts and death by suicide than those who are not. This is likely due to external influences such as isolation, bullying and not feeling accepted.

Reminder of the acronym:

B asics (Analyse, Break the ice, Crisis support)

E Escalate if needed

F oster a dynamic

R espond

E Explore support options

E stablish action plan

Scenario

Atif has just come out of a team meeting discussing plans for the next stage of the business, he looks visibly distressed and agitated. He is normally quite upbeat however recently he has seemed a bit down.

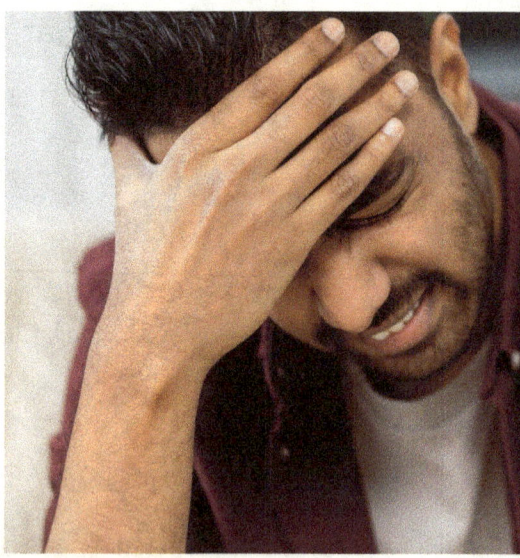

You approach him and he discloses that his wife has recently passed and that he's not doing well. They had been married for 7 years and her death was a shock. When you ask if he has had suicidal thoughts, he says he has made a plan to end his life.

How would you use the BEFREE model to respond to this situation?

How can mental health be promoted

Mind map of potential things that could be introduced or altered in the workplace to promote mental health - to be done individually

Resources

6 Core mental health standards

1 Produce, implement, and communicate a mental health at work plan.

2 Develop mental health awareness among employees.

3 Encourage open conversations about mental health and the support available when employees are struggling.

4 Provide employees with good working conditions and ensure they have a healthy work life balance and opportunities for development.

5 Promote effective people management through line managers and supervisors.

6 Routinely monitor employee mental health and wellbeing.

As a manager it's important to create the right culture within your team:

① Lead by example :

Actively encourage your team to adopt healthier working habits by working sensible hours, taking full lunch breaks, taking annual leave and resting after busy periods.

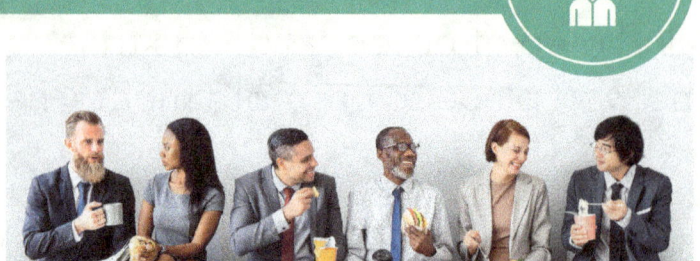

② Build your confidence on mental health :

Familiarise yourself with your organisation's mental health policies and practices and how staff can seek confidential advice and support.

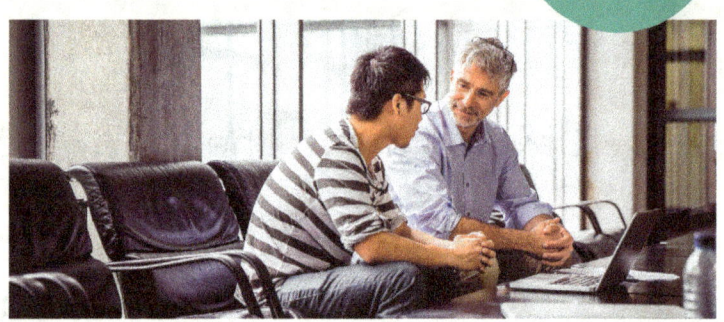

③ Normalise mental health :

Touch base regularly with your employees to check how they're getting on and think about what might be causing them stress. Create space for them to ask questions and raise issues, and give them permission to talk about home as well as work issues if they wish.

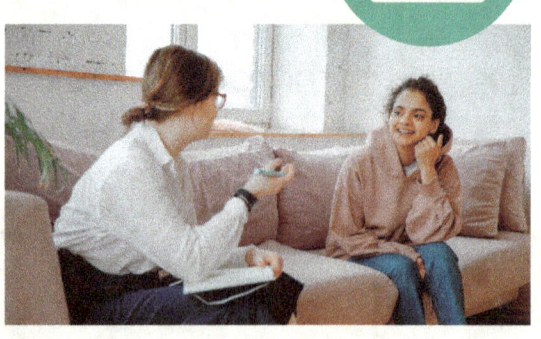

4 Take stock :

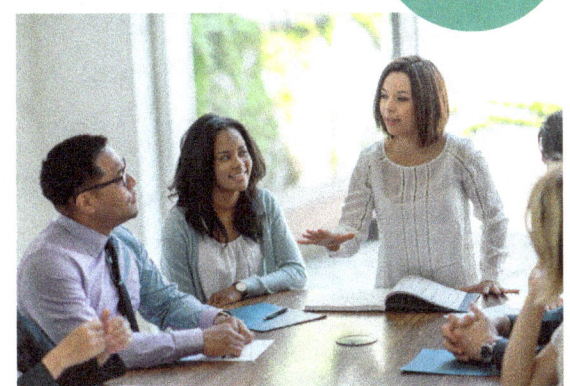

Include an agenda item at team meetings to discuss everyone's well-being together, and what factors are affecting this. A planning session can look at the issues in detail and develop a team action plan to address these. If the organisation runs a staff survey, this could form the basis of the discussion.

5 Be available for your staff :

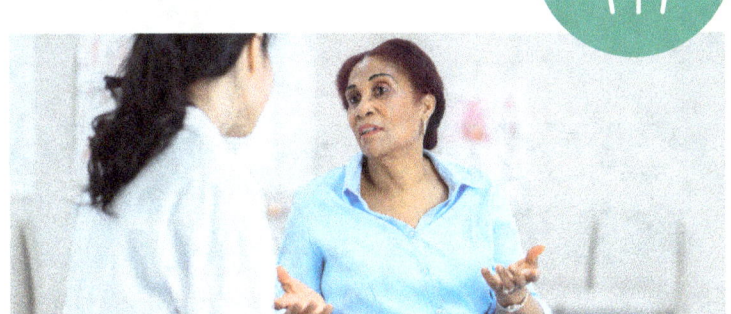

Regular one-to-ones and catch-ups can help to maintain good working relationships and build mutual trust.

6 Treat people as individuals :

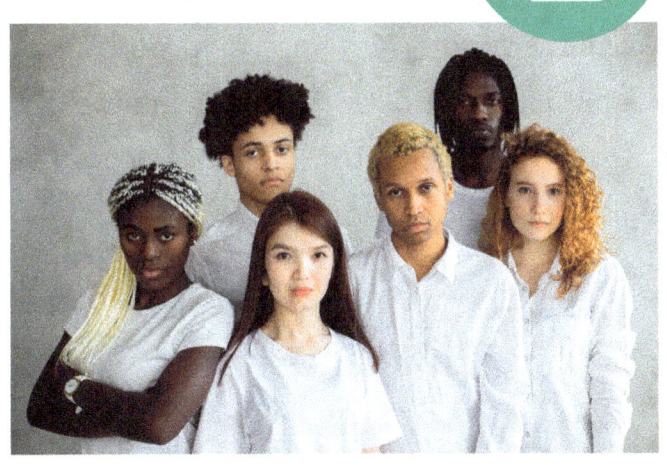

Treat employees with respect, praise good work, offer support if there are skills gaps, and try to use a coaching style of management. Ask for feedback about the support you provide and what support they need to help them achieve their goals.

Embed employee engagement :

Promote a culture of open dialogue and involve employees in decisions about how the team is run and how they do their job. Make sure employees understand their role in the bigger picture and make clear their contribution to the organisation's vision and aims.

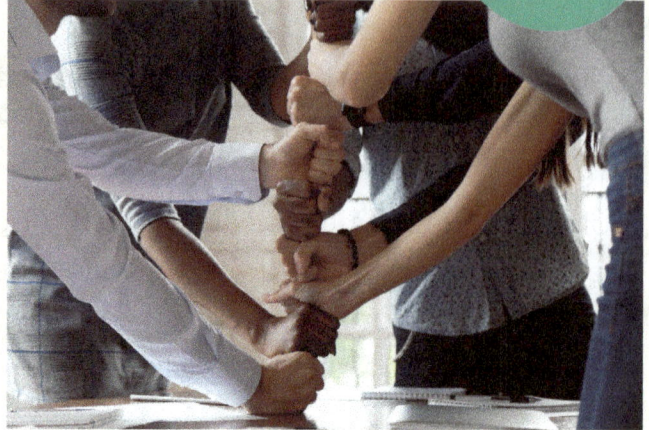

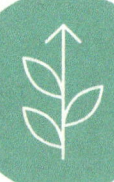 **Create opportunities for coaching, learning and development :**

Make sure employees are confident, well equipped and supported to enable them to do their job to a high standard. You can help them gain confidence and skills by developing and rewarding their capabilities and by being available for regular work-related conversations as well as providing formal training.

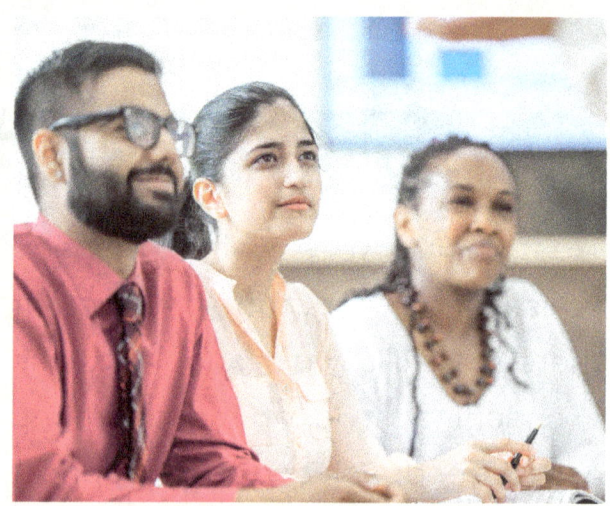

⑨ Promote positive work relationships :

Support a culture of teamwork, collaboration and information-sharing, both within the team and across the organisation, and model these positive behaviours to staff.

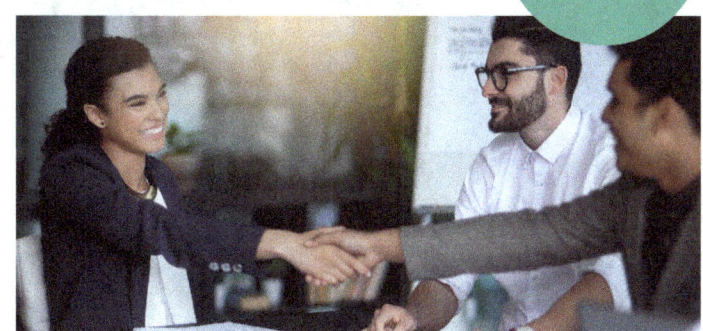

⑩ Raise awareness :

Managers are in a great position to challenge stigma and prejudice throughout the organisation and to get mental health on the agenda with senior leaders.

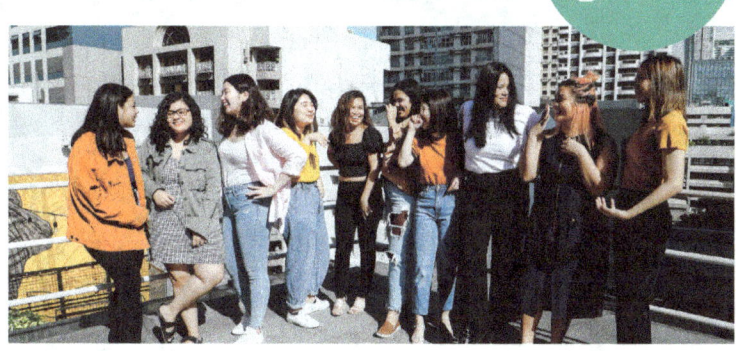

Dealing with Worries

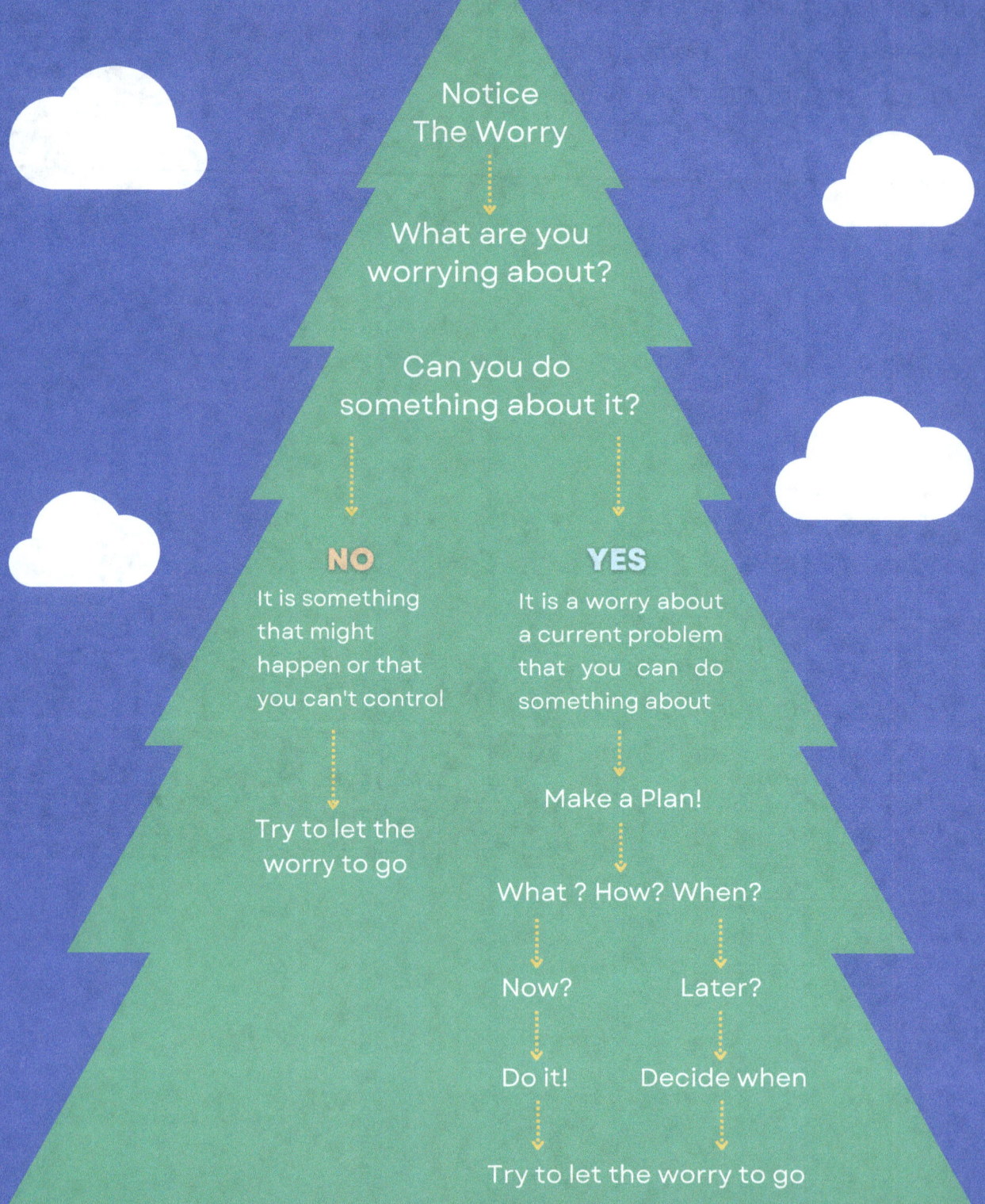

Notice The Worry

What are you worrying about?

Can you do something about it?

NO

It is something that might happen or that you can't control

Try to let the worry to go

YES

It is a worry about a current problem that you can do something about

Make a Plan!

What ? How? When?

Now?   Later?

Do it!   Decide when

Try to let the worry to go

Our mind and body

- Environment
- Situation

1
- Thought
- Mind

2
- Emotion
- Mood

3
- Physical
- Body

4
- Behaviour
- Action

Thought catching

Situation	
Emotion	
Thought	
Supporting Evidence	
Counter Evidence	
Alternative Thought	

Situation	
Emotion	
Thought	
Supporting Evidence	
Counter Evidence	
Alternative Thought	

Situation	
Emotion	
Thought	
Supporting Evidence	
Counter Evidence	
Alternative Thought	

Worries

Breaking down the things that worry you can help you deal with them better.

What are you worried about?

What are you worried about this? (Initial thoughts and feelings)

How can you reframe this situation?
For example, ' I wish I could do this ' can be " How can I do this".
This helps us look at things from a different perspective.

What are the different ways you can deal with this?

The calmer you are, the cleaner you think.

Start small, think about how you could be more optimistic.

Then think of other solutions. If there isn't a clear solution, break it down into how and when this happened, then work backwards.

Thoughts after reflection. Are you feeling more optimistic?

ETHOS

We aspire for mental health to be transformed and for the stigma surrounding it to be abolished. This book aims to inspire people to learn more about mental health and wellbeing and feel comfortable working with mental health professionals in order to look after themselves.

We hope to inform individuals how to look after their physical health: eat healthily, exercise more and avoid toxins.

We want to assist in making mental health and wellbeing improvement simple and easy for everyone. The more you can learn about the mind, the better quality of life you will exhibit.

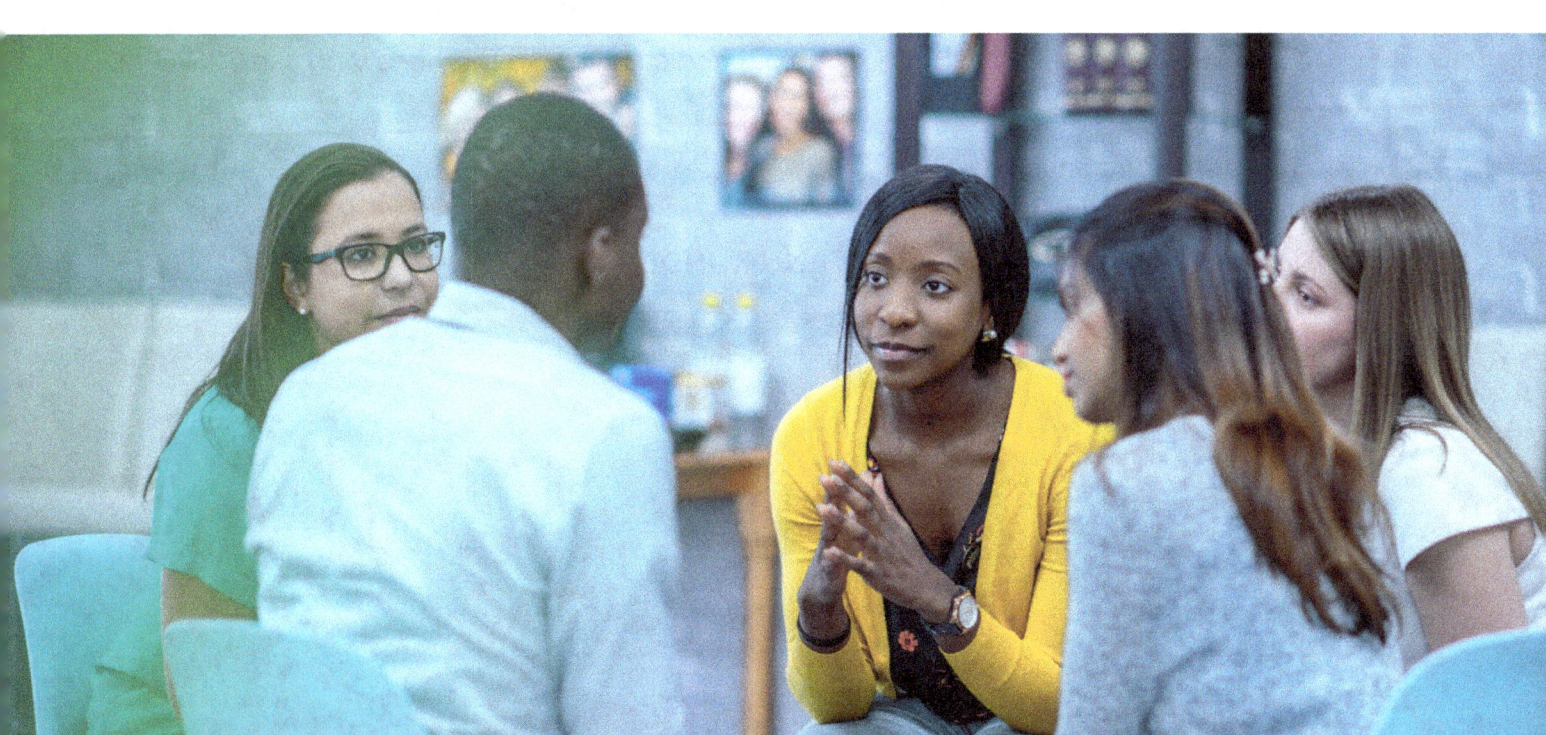

ABOUT THE BE FREE CAMPAIGN

The Be Free Campaign is an innovative award-winning mental health charity. Aiming to help people help themselves, improve their mental health, quality of life and improve access to health services. We are a registered charity committed to giving people the tools they need to look after their mental health and promote wellbeing within themselves and beyond. Supported by the National Lottery Fund and recognised by Rt. Hon. Boris Johnson - Prime Minister.

We work to improve mental health outcomes through sessions and workshops in schools, communities and lots more. Teaching about the world of mental health, preventative medicine, and improving access to mental health services. We work with celebrities and influencers, trying to promote positive mental health and to educate the public on what mental health actually is, as well as the various ways in which they can help to support the movement.

We live in a world where mental health is not given the attention it deserves. Mental health is something that everyone has and it is something we all have a right to look after. A lack of education, stigmatisation and critically underfunded services have led to the difficult circumstances that we see today. Our mission aligns with the nation and the wider world, by educating people about mental health and how they can best support it, we make sure to improve the way forward. We work to improve how the world looks at mental health. We work to normalise mental health by shouting out and standing up for those who can't. It's time to change. It's time to be free.

Break the stigma and Save Lives

SHANTANU KUNDU

FOUNDER/DIRECTOR
BE FREE CAMPAIGN

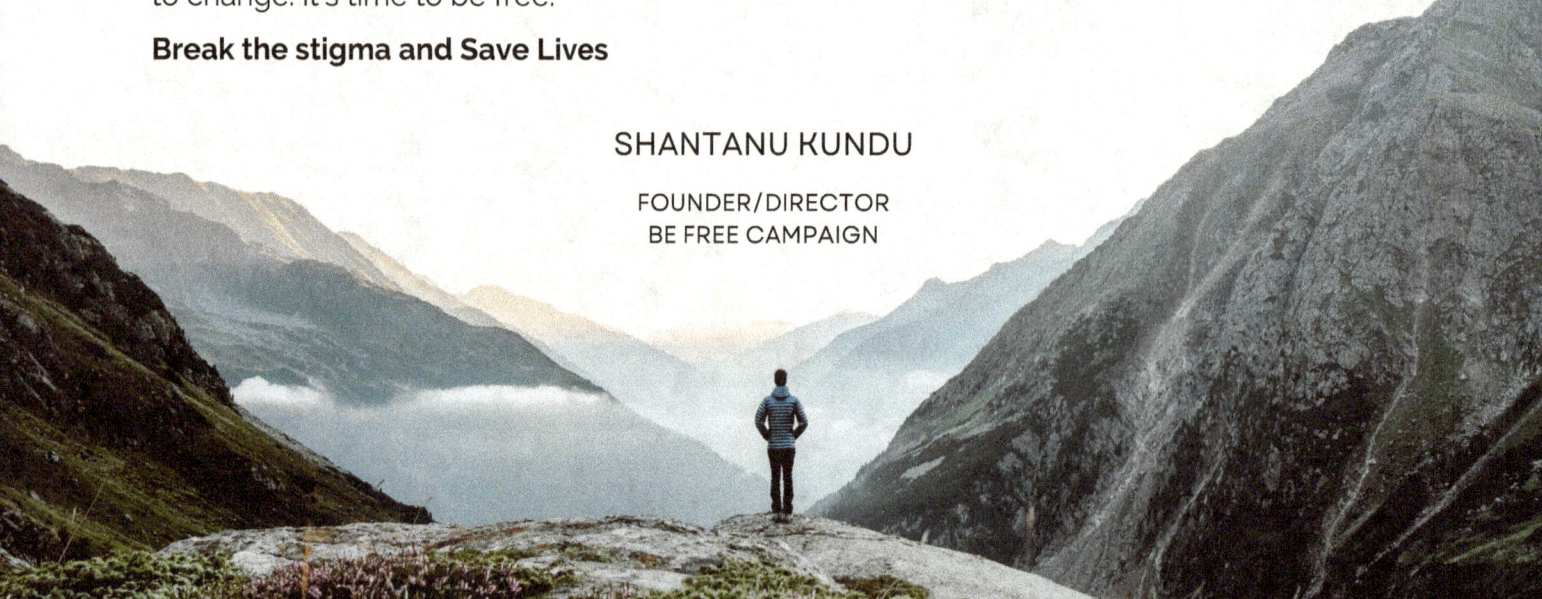

TRANSFORMING LIVES THROUGH TRANSFORMING MINDS

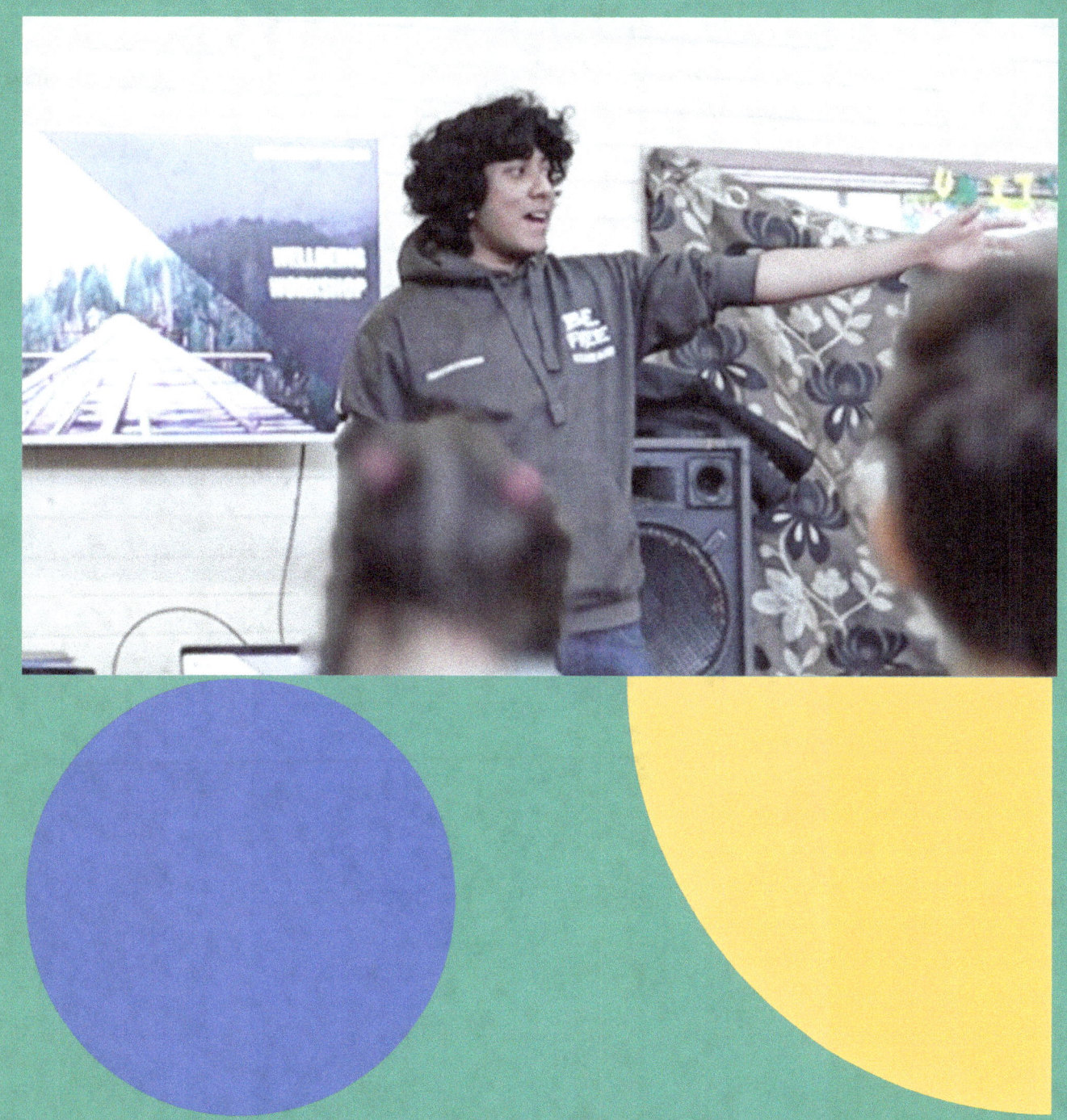

1
Wellbeing

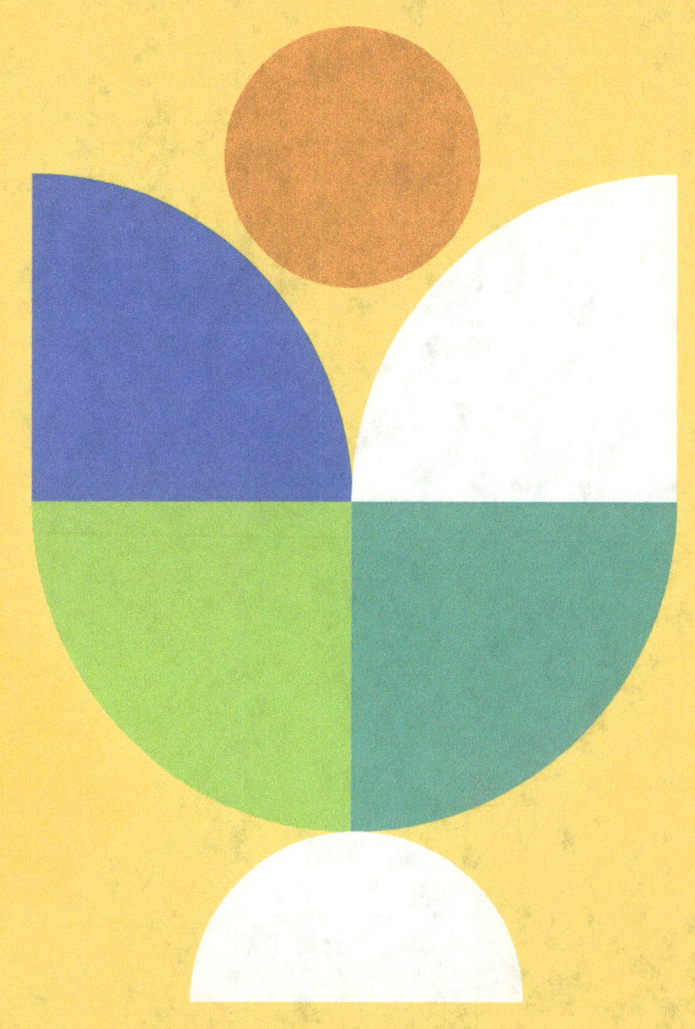

What is Wellbeing?

Wellbeing doesn't have a specific meaning. The Oxford English dictionary defines it as " the state of being comfortable, healthy, or happy." but it is much more diverse than these three words.

Mental wellbeing is different to mental health. Mental health regards our long term feelings - most mental health conditions require symptoms to be shown for several weeks. The distinction is that you can have poor mental health but good mental wellbeing (and vice versa). For example, you could be diagnosed with a mental health condition (technically poor mental health), yet still feel fine at that moment - good mental wellbeing.

Mental wellbeing and mental health are closely linked through things like resilience, coping ability and our hard work, which directly result in our wellbeing, but are partly determined by our mental health.

Although the concept of Wellbeing can be broad and hard to pinpoint, it generally encompasses how a person feels, functions and manages life. In simpler terms, positive wellbeing can be described as judging life positively and feeling good in day-to-day life. Wellbeing is a part of all our lives, and learning to look after our wellbeing can be one of the most useful tools a person can learn to lead a healthy life. Here is why...

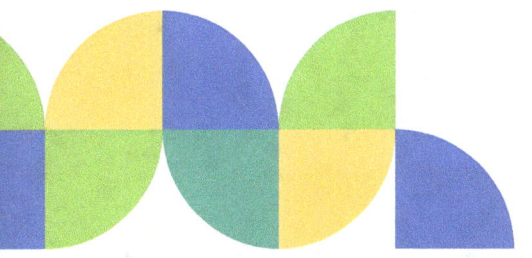

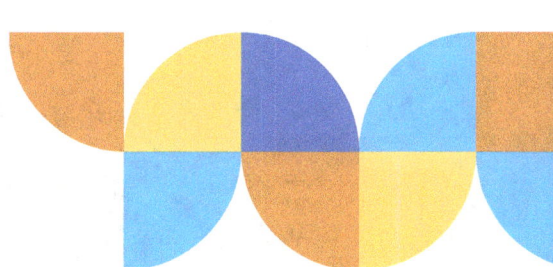

Why is wellbeing important?

Wellbeing is influenced by lots of different factors; some that are controllable and others that are not. Even if we can't influence some parts of our wellbeing, (e.g. illness, job, etc.) we can definitely affect our outlook on it, as well as become better at using tools to help it, which work together to build resilience! Improving our wellbeing can help in lots of unexpected ways. Creating positive methods and outlooks can help to view past experiences in a more realistic light, as well as preparing us mentally to successfully tackle future problems and achieve our goals. Improving our wellbeing can help us right now by changing perspectives on our thoughts and experiences. By improving our mental and physical wellbeing we can feel healthier and more in charge of our own life. We have the power to impact our own wellbeing. Working on our wellbeing isn't instant nor is it a key to unlocking ultimate happiness, but it is a step in the right direction. We can all implement small changes to get the best out of our lives. At the end of the day we only get one life so lets make it worth living!

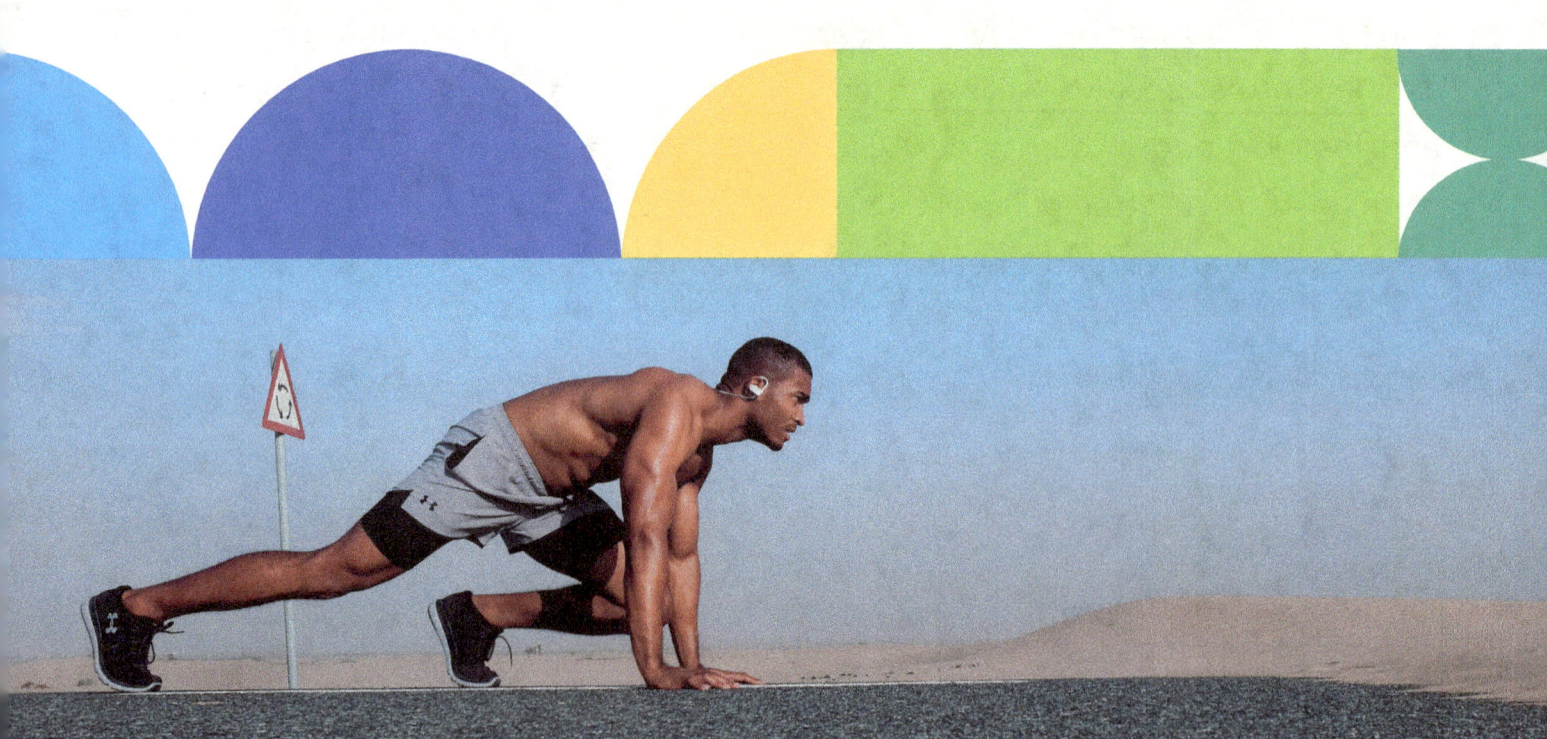

7 ways to wellbeing

We at The Be Free Campaign have developed seven key concepts which are pivotal in maintaining positive wellbeing in our lives. The seven concepts below are essential to helping foster positive wellbeing and allowing us to maintain positive mental health. You will see a marker in each of the tools throughout this booklet labelling which of the 7 ways to wellbeing it corresponds to.

CONNECT

EXERCISE

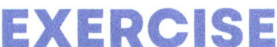
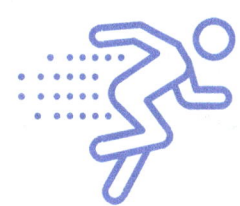

GIVING

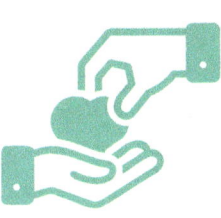

DIRECTION

TRYING OUT

REFLECTION

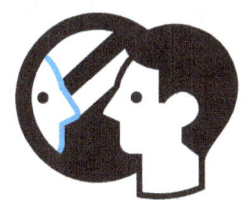

EMOTIONAL AWARENESS

Connect

Connecting refers to building strong relationships with people who can allow us to share our feelings and feel understood. These relationships can allow us to share positive experiences as well as to be able to receive and give emotional support.

Exercise

Being active releases positive neurotransmitters (more about them later), which can help us feel good. Having a positive connection with the outside can help us feel more connected and less lonely. Lastly, it can reduce stress and help us recover from mental health conditions.

Giving

Giving to someone else or to yourself can help improve our wellbeing in lots of ways! We can have an increased sense of purpose, positivity and it also exercises our ability to connect with others.

Direction

The direction in our lives is very important. Being able to set short and long-term goals gives us a very important sense of accomplishment which can help improve our mood and wellbeing.

Trying Out

Trying new things can be a really good way to improve our wellbeing. Learning a new skill or hobby can help us to build a greater sense of self-esteem and purpose from doing what we enjoy. It can be a great avenue for meeting new people and making new connections too!

Reflection

Being reflective of our own thoughts and emotions can give us a great insight into why we feel the way we feel. We can learn from our experiences which can help us reduce negative emotions and moods as well as help us on our way to being our best selves.

Emotional Awareness

Being aware of how we feel throughout the day and trying to do things that foster positive moods and emotions is very important for our wellbeing. Doing healthy things which impact our mood positively can assist in improving our wellbeing overall.

REFLECTION TRACKER

GOAL FOR THE WEEK:

	MON	TUE	WED	THU	FRI	SAT	SUN
EXPERIENCES:							
EMOTIONS:							
THOUGHTS:							

OVERALL THOUGHTS FOR THE WEEK...

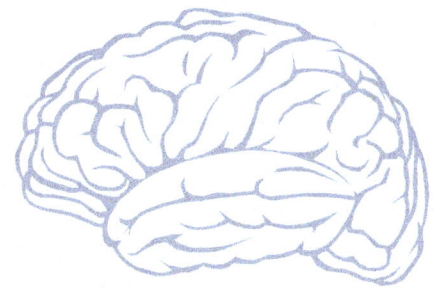

2
Day-to-day wellbeing

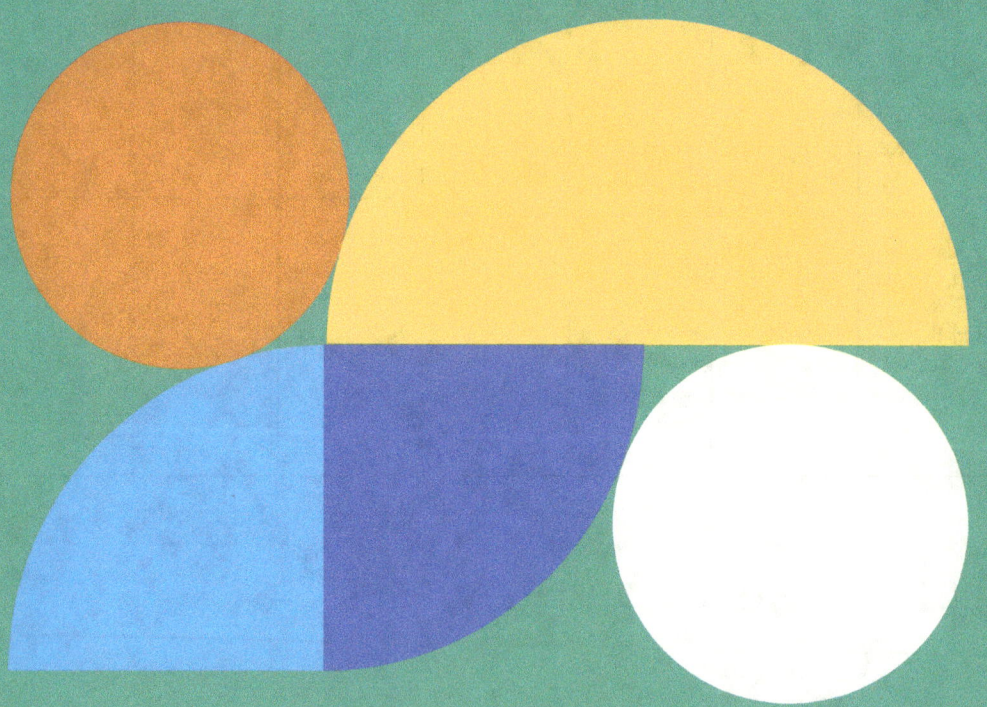

This section is aimed at giving you some tools to maintain your wellbeing. We will explore how to keep your body and mind healthy to protect your wellbeing. Firstly, we will investigate how our body impacts our wellbeing and the best ways we can keep our mind clean. Secondly, we will look into how we can keep our mind engaged and healthy. Hopefully, this section will give you some helpful protective tools that can be used to help keep your mental health positive.

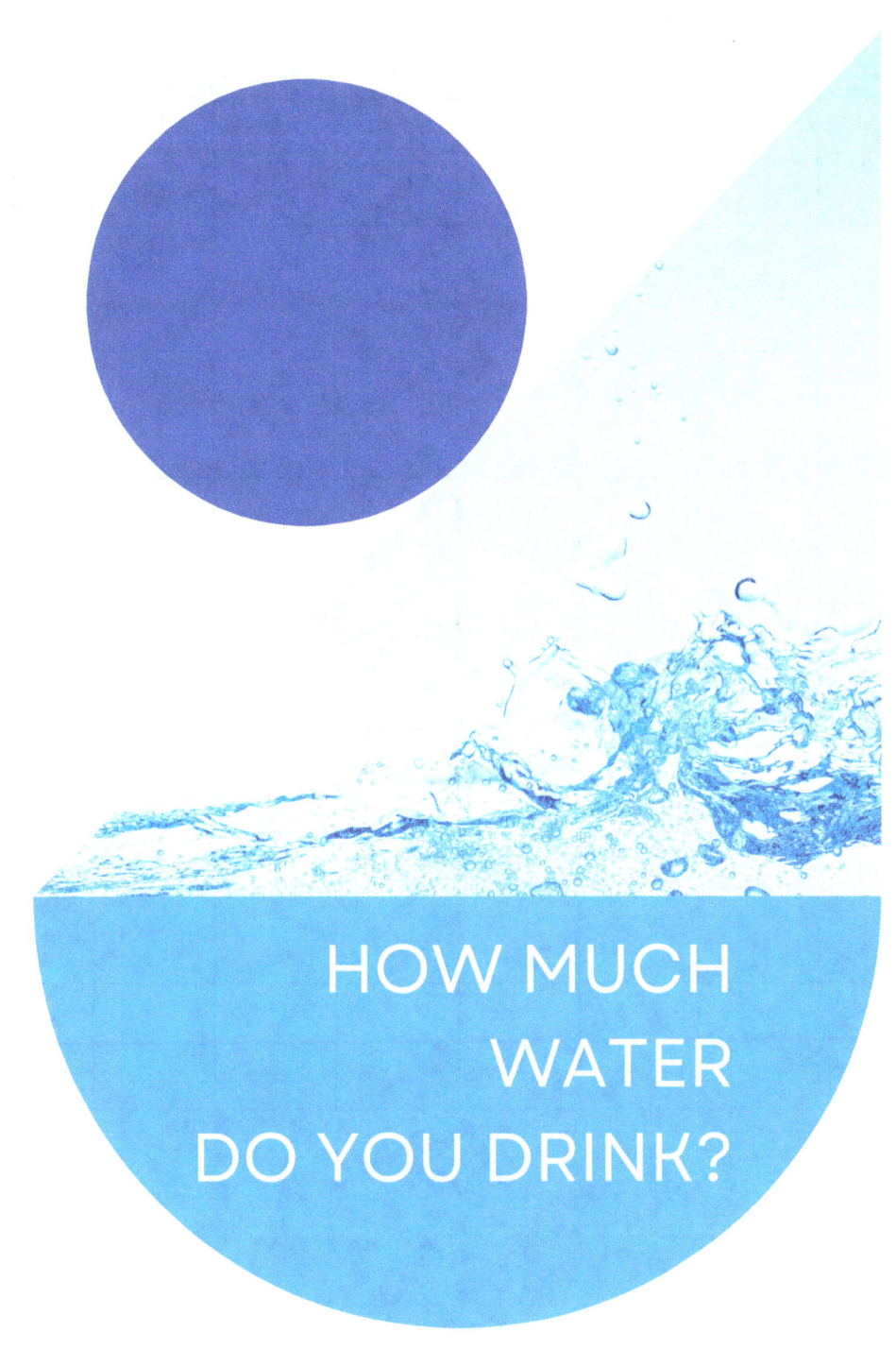

HOW MUCH
WATER
DO YOU DRINK?

WATER TRACKER

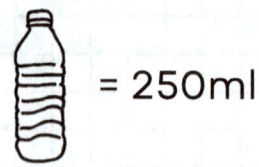 = 250ml

(RECOMMENDED WATER INTAKE)									
	🍶	🍶	🍶	🍶	🍶	🍶	🍶	🍶	🍶
MON									
TUE									
WED									
THU									
FRI									
SAT									
SUN									

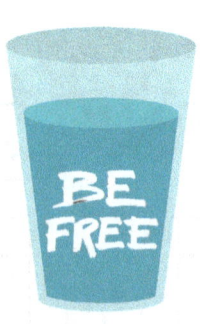

Water

Drinking the right amount of water is important for lots of reasons! Staying hydrated can help us stay both physically and mentally healthy. Your ideal daily water intake depends on lots of factors, but generally 2-3 litres (8-12 glasses) of water is a good amount to aim for.

WHAT ARE THE BENEFITS OF DRINKING WATER?

- Helps improve mood

- Delivers oxygen throughout the body – water makes up 90% of blood content!

- Boosts skin hydration and condition

- Important in neurotransmitter and hormone production

- Aids in digestion

- Maintains blood pressure

- Helps in breathing – airways are restricted by dehydration

- Prevents kidney damage

- Boosts performance during exercise

- Helps in serotonin production

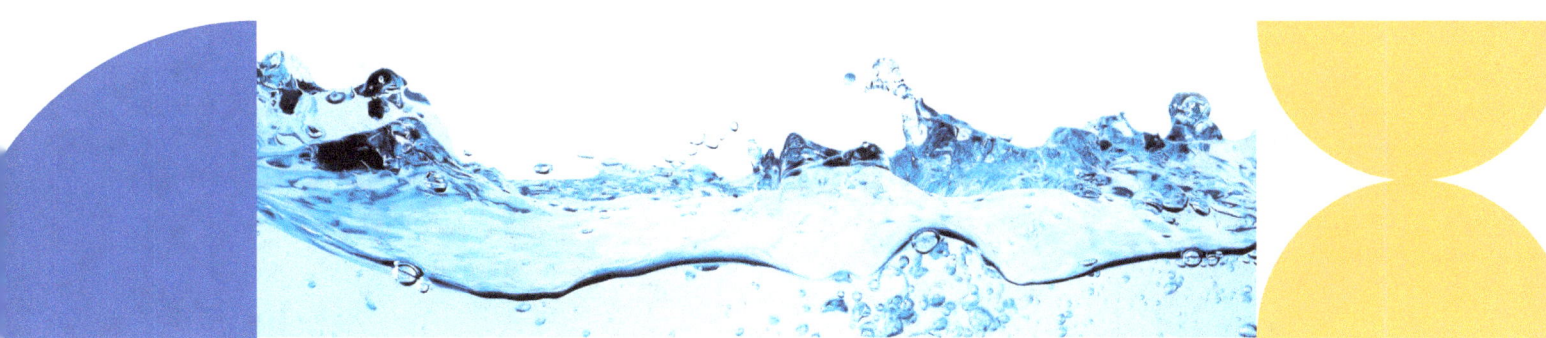

Serotonin

Wait. What is serotonin?

Serotonin is a neurotransmitter (a molecule that helps your brain communicate) that is involved in lots of processes but here are some of its most important functions – Primarily, serotonin helps to regulate mood and sleep but it also:

- Contributes in giving the brain energy – a lot of the chemical reactions in the brain need water to function

- Assists in combatting stress via reducing cortisol production

- Can assist in reducing panic attack symptoms by lowering heart rate, reducing the frequency of headaches, reducing muscle fatigue and weakness, and reduces light-headedness and fatigue

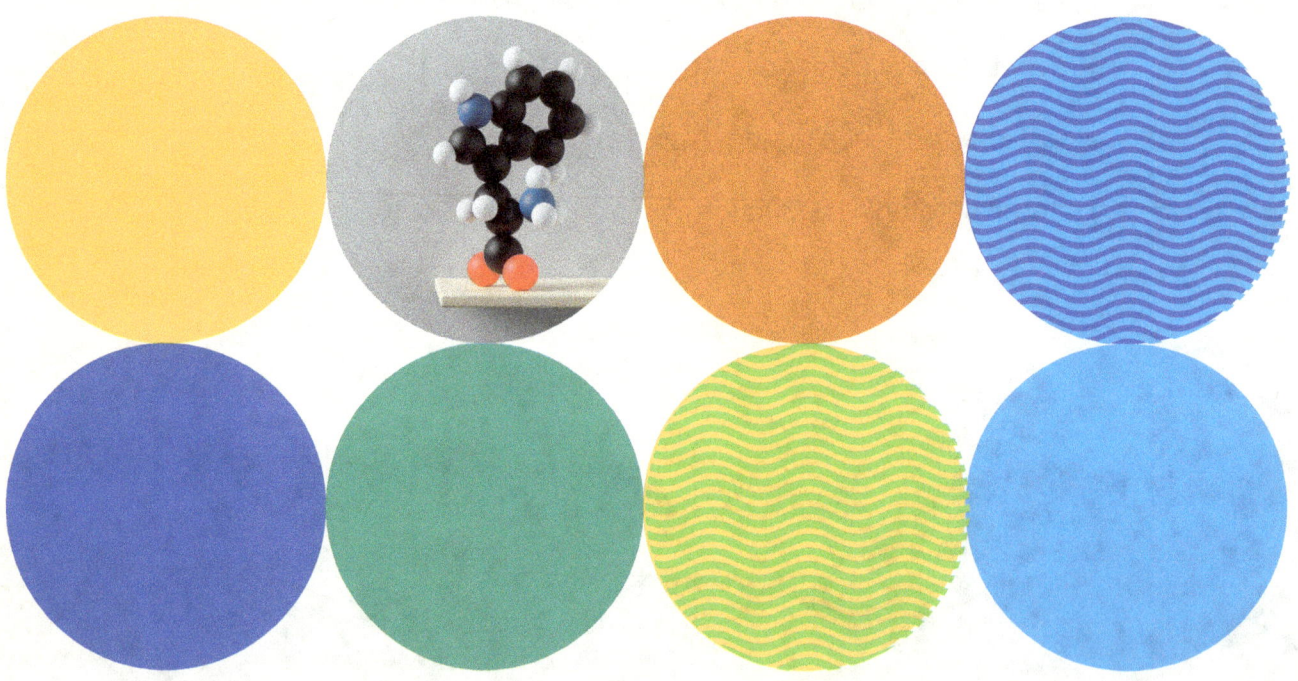

Eating

Eating is important for maintaining good physical and mental health. Our mind and body are influenced by the food we eat. Balancing our nutritional and vitamin intake can be essential in balancing our mental health and wellbeing. Having a healthy lifestyle includes having a healthy relationship with food too. Making sure you allow yourself to enjoy food without guilt is an important part of your mental and physical wellbeing. If you find yourself feeling upset about food, access support or ask for help by contacting your GP or mental health professional. Please see the "If you're not feeling too great" section for more information.

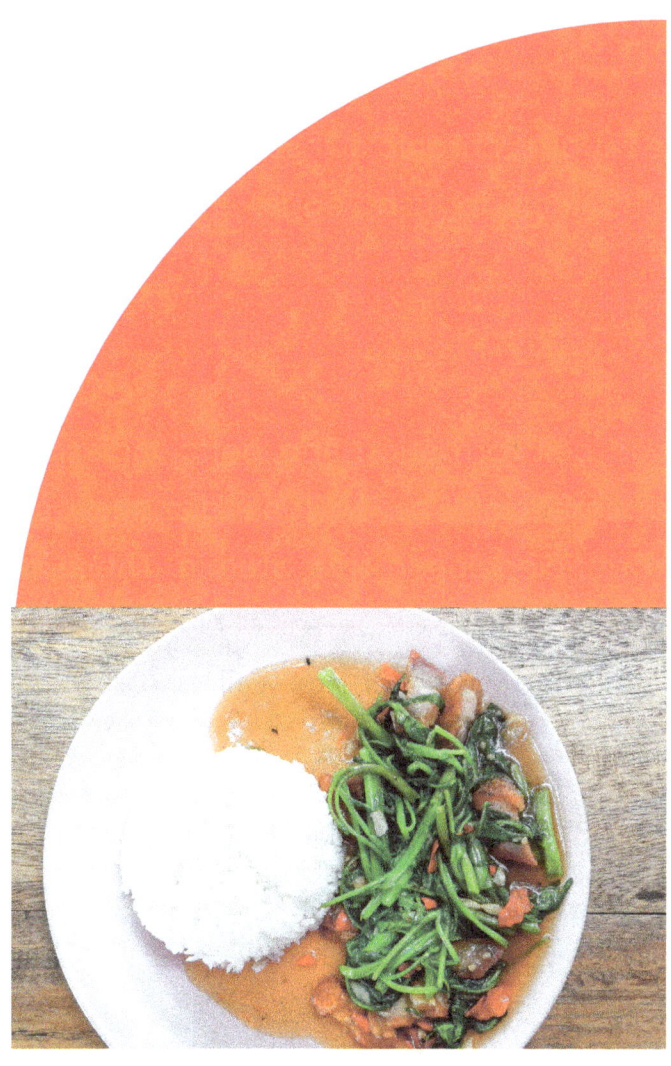
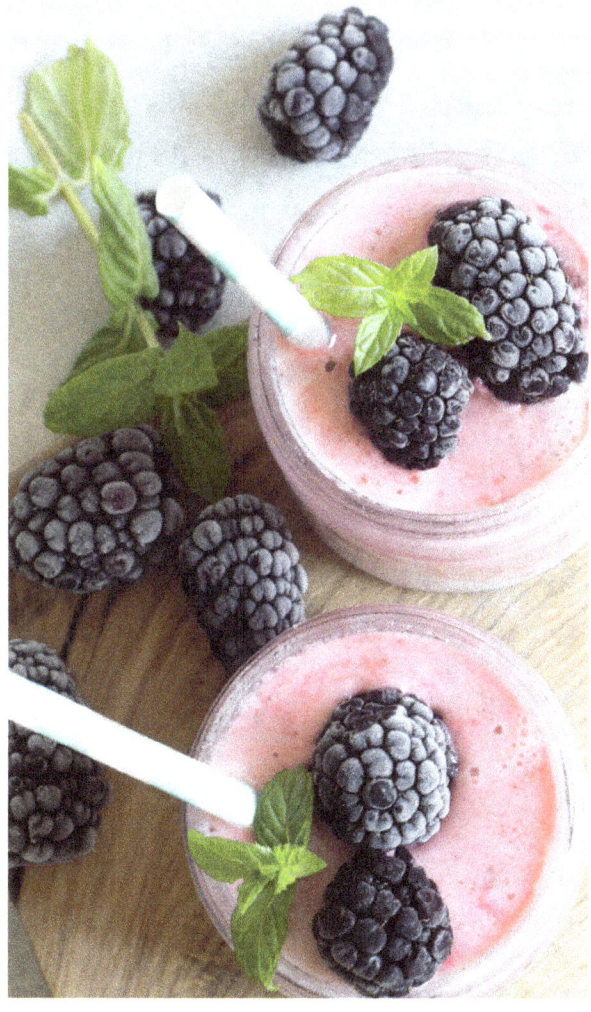

Vitamin B

These are a few examples of B-complex vitamins which are essential to mental health and wellbeing.

Vitamin B1

The brain uses this vitamin to help convert glucose or blood sugar into fuel, therefore, without it, the brain can rapidly run out of energy. This may lead to fatigue, irritability, anxiety, or depression. Foods that are rich in B1 include meats such as pork and beef, as well as non-meat alternatives such as sunflower seeds, whole grains and green peas.

Vitamin B1

Some symptoms of deficiency include fatigue, chronic stress, and depression. Foods that are highest in vitamin B5 include fish, eggs, avocados and mushrooms amongst other things.

Vitamin B12

This vitamin is important for red blood cell formation and deficiencies can cause mood swings, irritability and confusion, as well as dizziness and weakness. Some people are prone to deficiencies in this vitamin. These are some good natural sources to get some B12 back - milk, cheese, eggs, mussels and most meats alongside fortified soy milk as well as breakfast cereals.

Remember excessive alcohol intake can leave us with deficiencies in these vitamins.

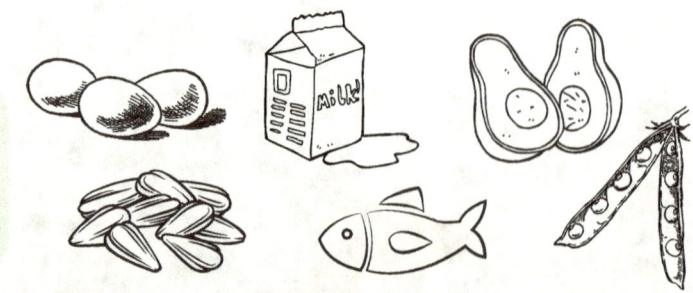

45

Other Vitamins and Minerals

Vitamin C (Ascorbic acid) ensures that skin, blood vessels, bones and cartilage are kept healthy. Deficiency in vitamin C can cause scurvy. The main sources of Vitamin C include citrus fruit, berries and brussels sprouts. It's best to get all the vitamins you need from a well-balanced diet. Speak to your doctor if you are worried and they can recommend supplements if needed.

Vitamin D is a really important essential nutrient for our body as it helps with the regulation of calcium and phosphate. Deficiency can lead to osteomalacia in adults and rickets in children. Our body can use sunlight to synthesise vitamin D, so during months of cloudy weather, we often don't get enough vitamin D. Supplements can help out here, speak to your doctor for more information.

Vitamin A can help with retinol which helps in low light vision, immune system strength and skin integrity. Vitamin E also helps maintain healthy skin and eyes, as well as aiding the immune system.

Other minerals like iron, calcium, magnesium and folic acid are really important for overall health. Issues in mood can be related to deficiencies in these various minerals so it is important you get yourself checked out by a family doctor if you need to!

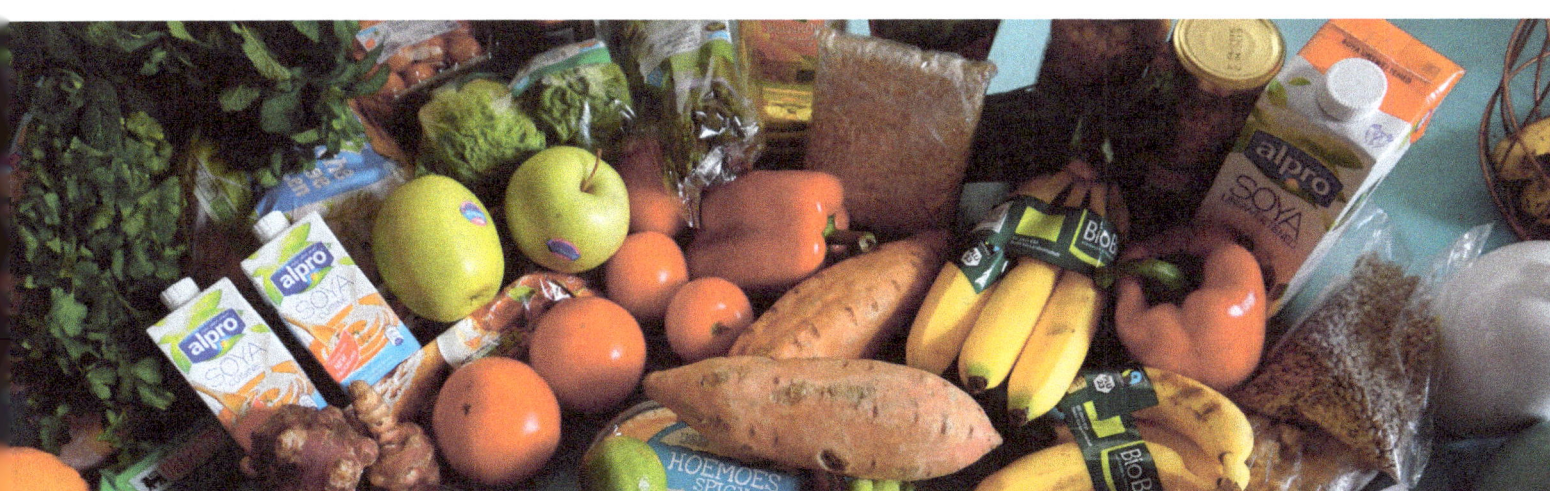

The Importance of a good diet

In order to help maintain good mental health, it is important that you eat a balanced diet. We need the foundations of a healthy diet to help us face our daily tasks.

Although it sounds cliché, you really do need your 5 a day of fruit and vegetables. Not only do they contain vitamins, minerals and plenty of antioxidants, but they also contain fibre. The role of fibre in our health comes to play when it's digested by our gut bacteria, who transfer all the benefits straight to us. These bacteria produce molecules that travel in our bloodstream and help improve things like our immunity and brain health. Scientists are even linking fibre with reduced rates of mental health conditions!

Having a balanced diet means eating a range of all foods. We don't just need the 'healthy' stuff, we need the other stuff too. Foods high in sugar and fat still have a place in our diet, and our brains are even hard-wired to enjoy them so don't beat yourself up if you treat yourself to a slice of cake every so often. However, that sugary breakfast can have an impact on your digestion and your cortisol levels (we will speak about this soon). When you have quick-acting processed sugary foods, you end up with a sugar crash. This can make you shaky, hungry, slow down your digestive system, increase weight gain and even make you more stressed.

When our brain lacks fuel, it can often leave us feeling irritable and easily annoyed. To avoid this, make sure you are getting your carbohydrates from whole grain sources, like brown pasta, rice or bread. These foods release their energy slowly into your bloodstream and stop you from getting those highs and lows you might get from eating white carbs or sugary snacks.

Making sure you are eating enough protein will guarantee yourself the perfect amount of amino acids to help your body make essential neurotransmitters, like dopamine and serotonin, that make us feel happy. Good sources of protein include meat, fish and dairy, as well as plant sources like beans, pulses and nuts.
Lastly, reducing or eliminating habits such as alcohol, nicotine intake, refined sugars, and caffeine as much as possible can help you feel physically and mentally healthier.

Stress

At the most basic level, stress is our body's response to pressures from a situation or life event. What contributes to stress can vary hugely from person to person and differs according to our social and economic circumstances, the environment we live in and our genetic makeup.

Cortisol is a hormone you may have heard about, or never heard about at all. It is often called the stress hormone and carries out a variety of actions on the rest of your body. Sometimes this response can be helpful and appropriate to get us through situations. However, ongoing stress can become overwhelming and can have a tiresome effect on the body making us feel unable to cope.

Your immune system can be affected. The system that protects us from the world of bugs can go into excessive inflammation if you have too much cortisol. This means you can get sick easier and heal slower. A study from King's College London in 2016 showed that inflammation and this idea of chronic inflammation can actually increase symptoms from depression, as well as decrease the efficacy of treatments. Trying to decrease stress may lead to a lot of improvements around the body.

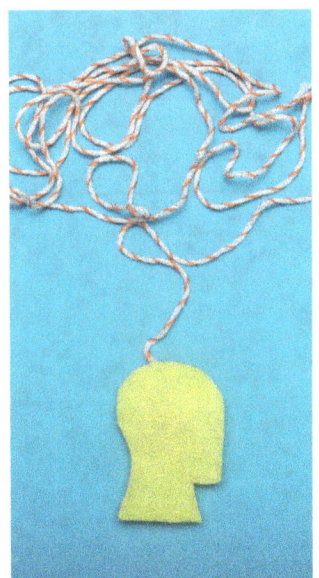

Signs of stress can include...

- Emotional changes: depression, anxiety, anger, irritability, feeling overwhelmed,

- Behavioural changes: changes in appetite, procrastinating, avoiding responsibilities, increased use of alcohol, drugs/cigarettes

- Bodily changes: headaches, upset stomach, chest pain, trouble sleeping, high blood pressure

There are a few ways in which stressed people can manage their lifestyles for better wellbeing. Follow this toolkit step-by-step and take your time! Change takes time.

Stress busters

Talk to a friend or colleague about your feelings

Find family or friends who can help advise you on managing your stress. Saying your problems out loud will help you take some control back to improve your life. This will help you acknowledge the causes of your stress and together with a trusted individual you can formulate a plan to find practical solutions, realistic expectations and goals.

Review your lifestyle

The chances are you are taking on too much in your life. By reviewing your lifestyle, there is the possibility to hand some responsibility for things to others, telling the appropriate people you are struggling (e.g. your academic advisor or boss) and prioritising the important things. Organisation skills are key for this. Produce a timetable or a list of things in order of importance for the week so you do one thing at a time.

Build up supportive relationships

If your stress is related to education or work, a good way to alleviate the stress is to build up a support network through a leisurely activity. Joining a leisure centre or volunteering for a charity will help to take your mind off the stress and will improve your mood drastically.

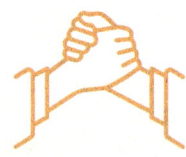

Eat healthily

Healthier eating habits will firstly reduce the risk of certain diseases such as diabetes and heart disease, but there is also evidence that shows healthier eating to be associated with a better general mood. This can help generate positive feelings of wellbeing if we eat healthy foods with the correct vitamins, minerals and nutrients. Cutting down on alcohol and smoking which can cause worsened anxiety and aggression will reduce the tense feelings associated with stress. Don't forget water as well! You can read all about this in more detail in the Diet and Water sections.

Exercise

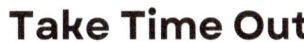

Taking a daily walk around the park or joining the gym helps improve wellbeing as these activities release endorphins which improve general mood. At the minimum, 15-20 minutes of exercise a day has proven to make a difference. You can find some simple, effective exercises in the next section of this handbook

Take Time Out

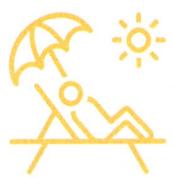

It is important to have you time! Take time out to relax and take care of yourself. This could be in the form of a relaxing bath with music and face masks or watching a few episodes of your favourite program for a few hours at the end of each day. This will allow time for self-reflection and positive thinking which can alleviate stress levels after a busy day..

Be Mindful

Mindfulness is a new technique which is being researched and proven to work well. It helps reduce the effects of stress such as anxiety and depression and changes this into positive mental thinking. Refer to the Mindfulness and Meditation sections in the handbook.

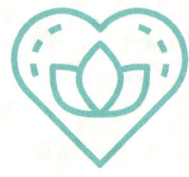

Sleep

Stressed individuals can have trouble getting to sleep due to symptoms of stress like tension and anxiety. Reducing caffeine intake and avoiding bright lights as you are going to bed may help you fall asleep easier. Most people will be stressed about what they have to do next. To reduce this, writing a list for the next day before you go to sleep may ease anxiousness about getting things done as you have a plan! You can refer to the sleep section of this handbook for more information.

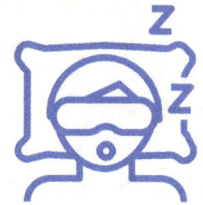

Look at things in perspective and do not be too hard on yourself! Writing down the positive things in your life that make you happy is a great way to look at things in perspective and focus on positive thinking. These changes will take time so try not to put pressure on yourself to not feel stressed overnight! If you need further help, seeking professional help would be the next step in feeling better about yourself again.

Exercise

Physical activity can hugely enhance our wellbeing by increasing our mental alertness, energy, sharpening memories and boosting sleep quality. This is particularly good for alleviating symptoms of stress such as anxiety and muscle tension. Physical activity also increases self-esteem, as exercise promotes chemical releases of endorphins in the brain which helps boost mood and makes us more relaxed. This is a simple but powerful medicine for better mental health.

You shouldn't overwork yourself and exercise too much. Adults are recommended to do around 5 hours a week of moderate exercise. The gym is not compulsory. Exercising can be in the form of walking, running, playing a sport, or home workouts.
It doesn't matter what your age or ability is, simple exercises done for only 15-20 minutes have evidently shown improvement to well-being!

Start with small goals, schedule exercise for times when energy is highest, focus on forms of exercise you enjoy (ex. a sport rather than the gym), be comfortable, reward yourself and find exercise buddies to make it more fun!
Getting started with a new thing can be hard when you struggle with your mental wellbeing. On the next page are 3 accessible exercises to incorporate into your daily lives.
Make sure the area around you is clear before you begin!

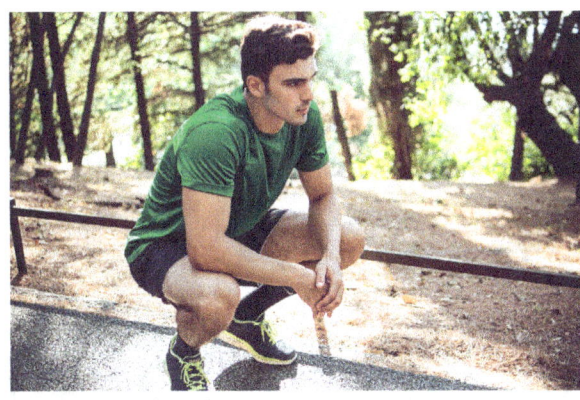 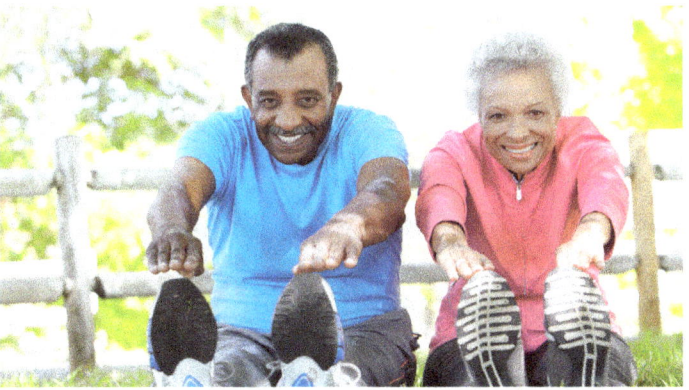

Exercises you can try!

5 wall/chair push-ups after every cup (of tea) (3 sets of 5-10 repetitions).

- Stand at arm's length from a wall/chair. Place the palm of your hands against the wall at chest level with your fingers pointing upwards.
- Keep your back straight, slowly bend your arms and keep your elbows by your side. Close the gap slowly between you and the wall/chair by pushing your chest closer to the wall.
- Slowly return to the start and repeat.

Mini-squats after each episode you watch (5-10 times)

- Find a chair for stability if required. Rest your hands on the back of the chair and stand with your feet shoulder-width apart.
- Slowly bend your knees as far as you can, keeping them facing forward towards the chair. Keep your back straight at all times.
- Gently come up to standing and clench your buttocks as you do so.

Bicep Curls after every snack (3 sets of 5 curls with each arm)

- Hold a pair of light weights and stand shoulder-width apart. You can be as creative as you want with filled up water bottles, bags of sugar or cans of beans!
- Keep your arms by your side, slowly bend them until the weight in your hands reaches your shoulder.
- Slowly lower again and repeat

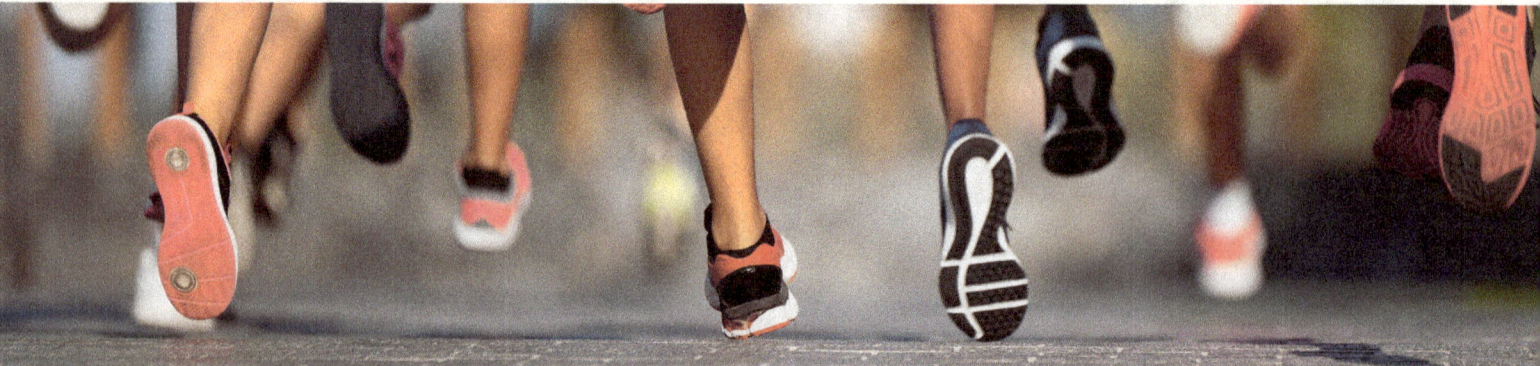

Yoga and its MYTHS

Yoga is translated as 'union'; it refers to disconnecting from the external world that can cloud our heads. Yoga aims to help our mental wellbeing by uniting body and mind to create peace.

Yoga can be used as a form of meditation and therapy which involves guiding the individual through breath work, meditation and movement to increase the sense of awareness and uplifting feelings. As yoga involves a light level of exercise and performing different poses and stretches, it is no wonder it is proven to have a positive affect on mental health, wellbeing and physical health.

When you're having to focus on holding a pose or breath work, it creates less time distracted with a chattering mind.

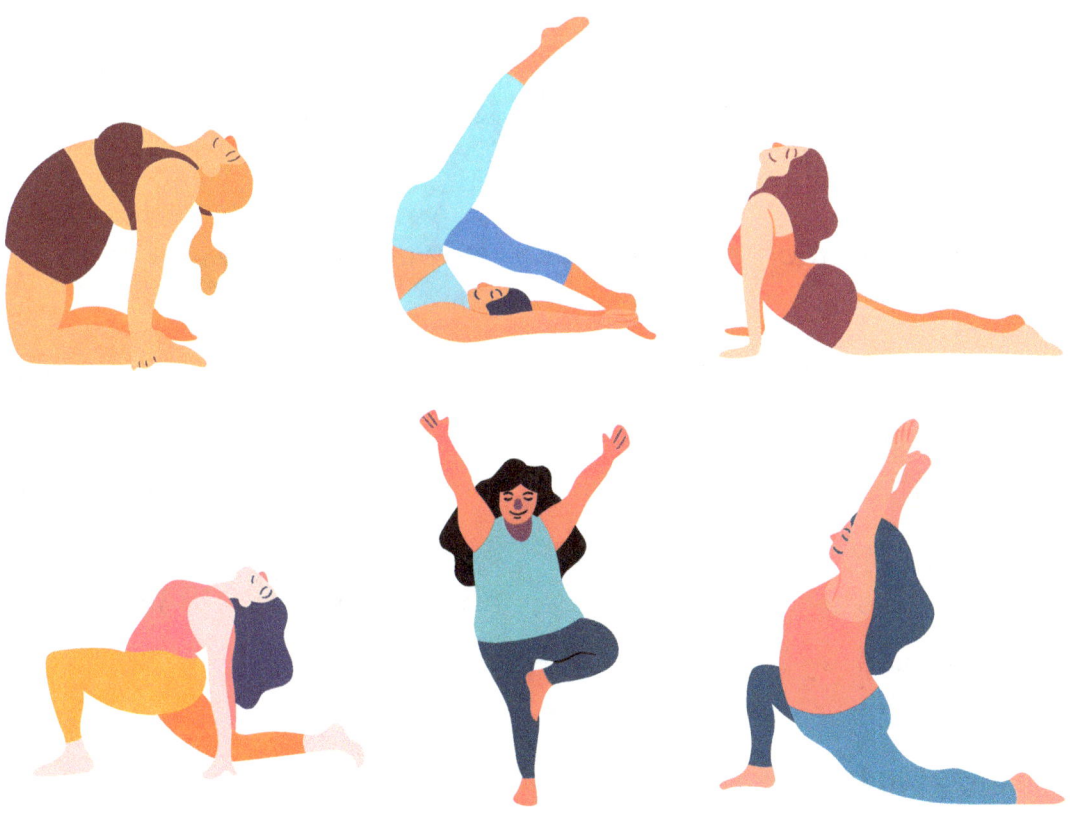

THERE ARE MYTHS ABOUT YOGA THAT CAN SOMETIMES PUT PEOPLE OFF:

You have to be super fit to do yoga

It is a hard physical exercise

It is only good if you're flexible

You're either good or bad at yoga

It just involves stretching and being quiet

BENEFITS OF YOGA:

Improves posture   Increases strength   Helps improve fitness

Lowers blood pressure   Improves balance   coordination   Reduces anxiety

Teaches relaxation techniques

Feel part of a community

THERE ARE DIFFERENT TYPES OF YOGA THAT CAN SUIT PEOPLE FOR ALL REASONS; HERE ARE A COUPLE:

Types of Yoga

1. Hatha- the foundation for all yoga – slower pace- restorative- good for beginners
2. Vinyasa- active class incorporating a range of poses flowing- fast-paced – more active
3. Hot yoga- any practice of yoga carried out in a heated room. Helps improve flexibility.
4. Ashtanga- poses and sequences carried out for longer help provide deep stretches and release tension.

Yoga is accessible from various resources, check out the resource page at the end of the book!

Routine

A routine is like a habit or sequence of activities that remain mostly constant on a daily basis. Having a routine makes us feel that we're in control and can reduce our stress levels. It can allow us to have better time management so we are able to allocate time to the things we really want to do. Having a routine helps us foster self-discipline, which can help us remain on track towards our goals and allows us to remain organised. It can also promote our organisation skills which can make our day more efficient and smoother. Fostering a routine involves creating a healthy work-life balance which ensures that you have the necessary time to complete your work and personal goals, as well as time to relax. Behavioural activation is a mental health treatment, which aims at combatting low mood by increasing your activity level and getting yourself back into a routine.

DO YOU HAVE A ROUTINE?

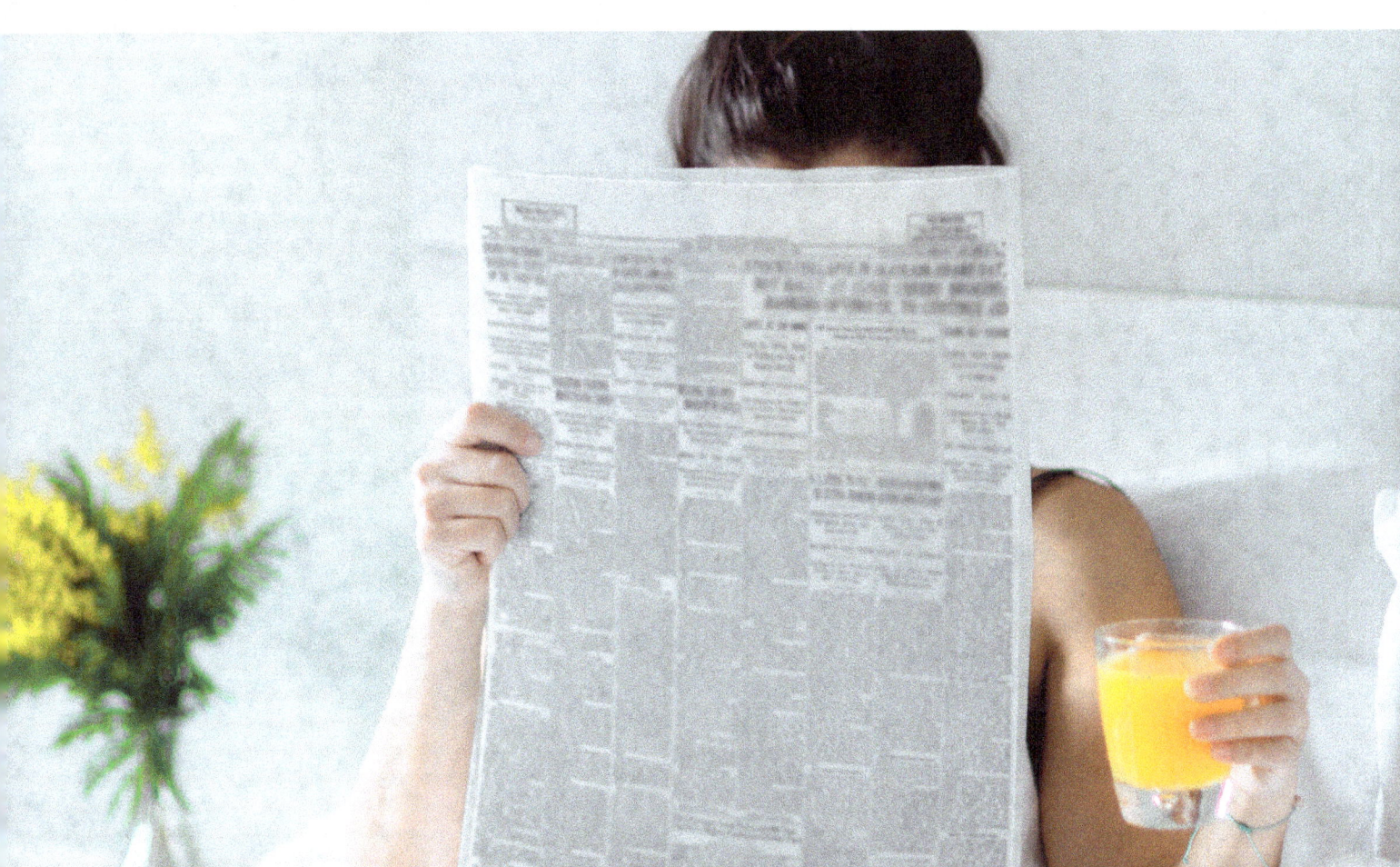

HOW TO BUILD A ROUTINE

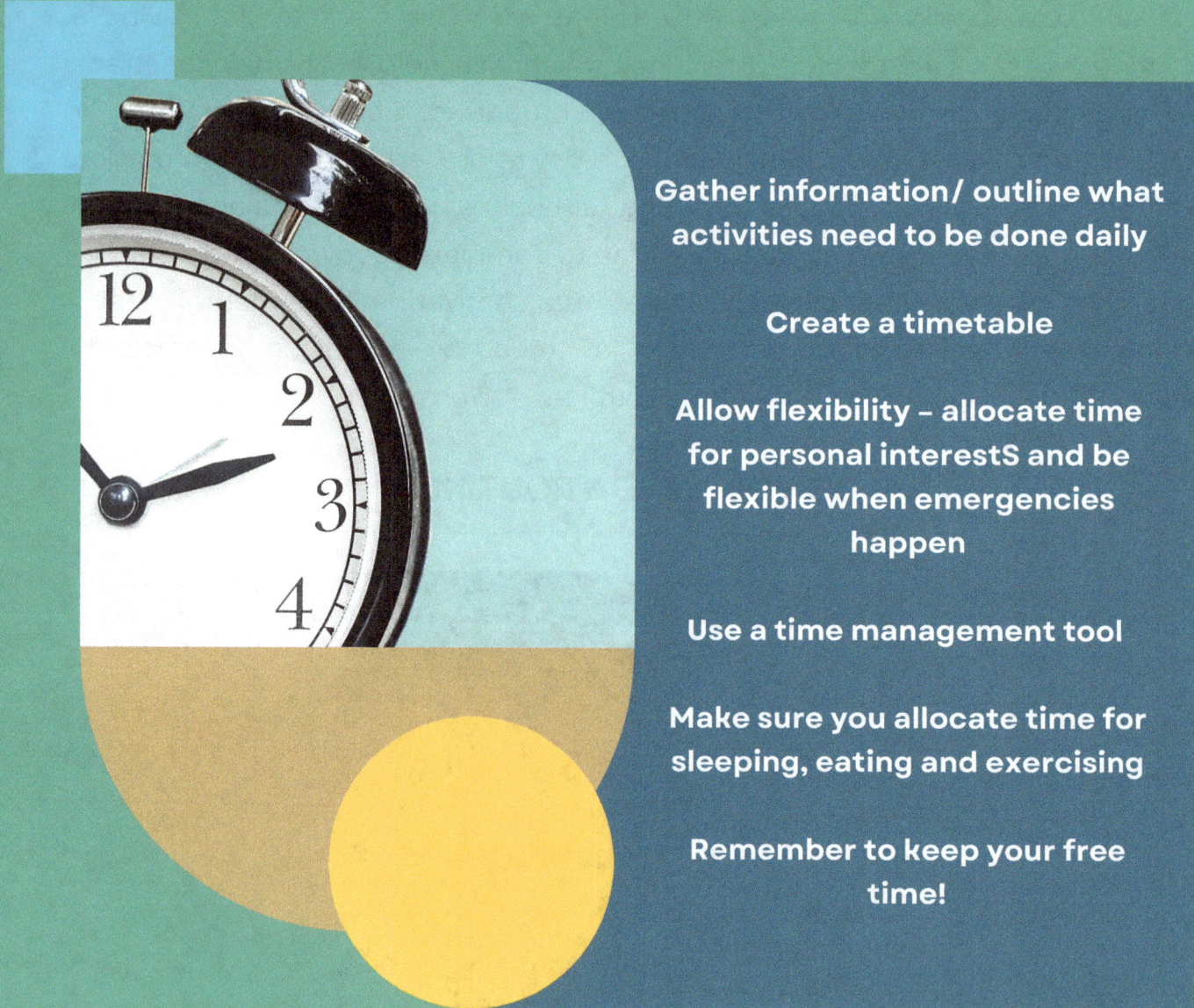

Gather information/ outline what activities need to be done daily

Create a timetable

Allow flexibility – allocate time for personal interestS and be flexible when emergencies happen

Use a time management tool

Make sure you allocate time for sleeping, eating and exercising

Remember to keep your free time!

Try using a to do list for the day or a diary. Both ways can be really helpful when trying to organise a day!

3
Mental Wellbeing

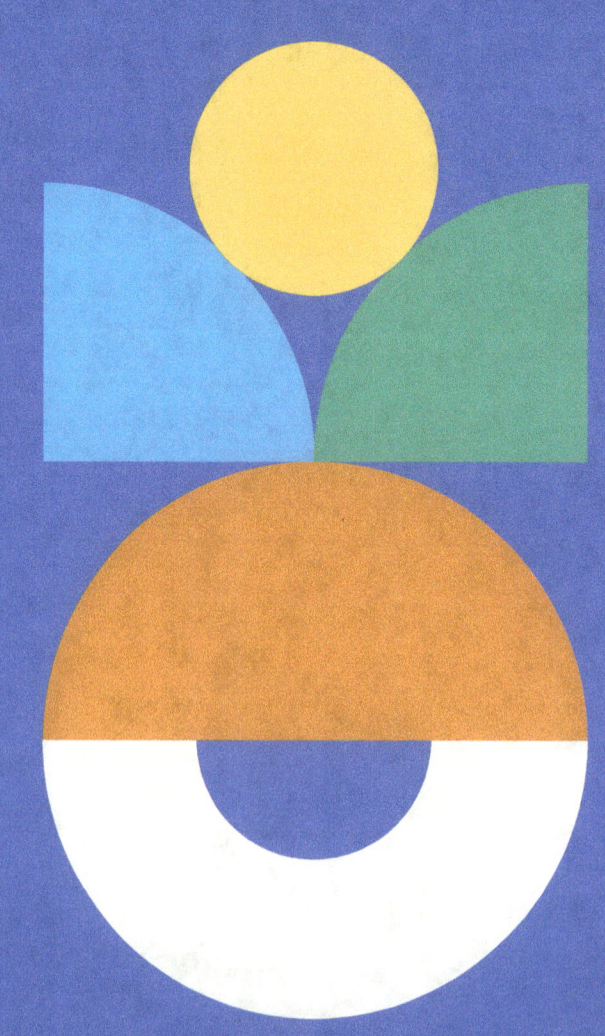

Gratitude

Gratitude is more than feeling thankful. Gratitude can be a deeper appreciation for someone or something that produces longer lasting positivity. It is the appreciation of what is valuable and meaningful to you and represents a general state of thankfulness or appreciation.

Gratitude can help someone feel more positive about their situation and relish a good experience. Gratitude has been shown to help our health, deal with adversity, and build strong relationships. People feel and express gratitude in multiple ways.

The significance of gratitude and the benefits it has on the individual:

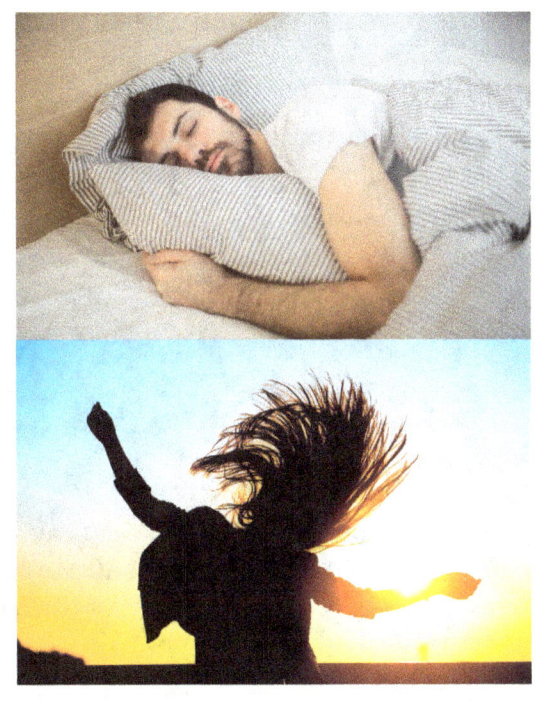

- Improves mood
- Better sleep
- Helps minimise stress
- Improves physical health.
- Improves psychological health.
- Enhances empathy and reduces aggression.
- Improves self-esteem

When things aren't going too well and everything feels a bit difficult it is important to take it one step at a time. Try starting off small with little daily reminders that you can repeat in your head. Try making a grateful reminder/saying that you can have for when things aren't going great. Give yourself some time on your own in the morning or evening reflecting on what you can be grateful for that day or practising your reminder.

Here are three exercises to help you practice gratitude:

1. Each day, think of 3 things you are grateful for. Nature. People. Community. Shelter. Creature comforts like a warm bed or a good meal. It's amazing what you notice when you focus on feeling grateful.

2. Start a gratitude journal. Making a commitment to writing down good things each day makes it more likely that you will notice good things as they happen.

3. Tell someone that you are grateful for them. This can be anyone from a partner to a cashier. Let them know that you are thankful for how they have treated you. You'd be surprised how it can help improve both of your days.

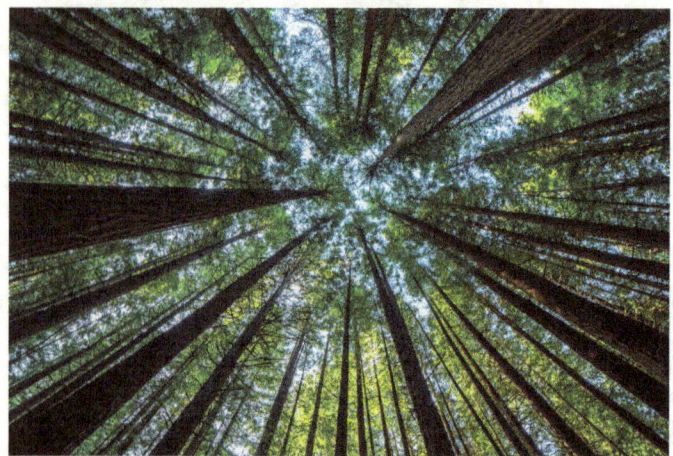

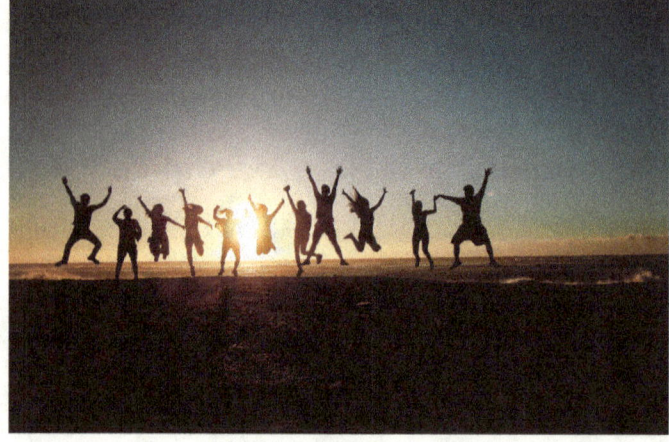

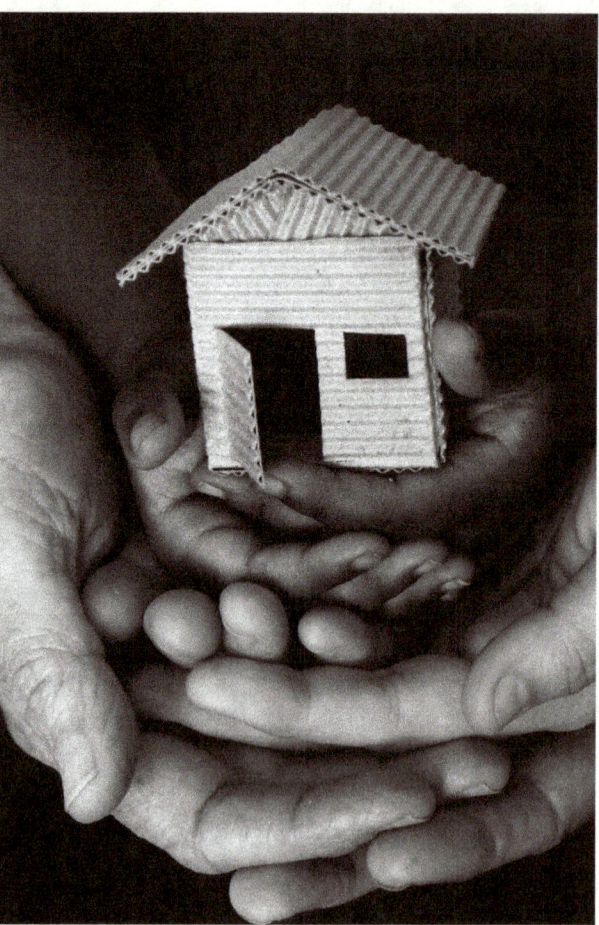

Disclosure

Disclosing your mental wellbeing, good or bad, to yourself, friends, family or others can be a great step forward towards promoting positive wellbeing. The act of disclosing your mental wellbeing to either yourself and/or others can have positive effects on the way you view, manage and interact with yourself. This section will teach you how to start this process...

Self

Getting to know your own mental health can really help you promote your own wellbeing. You can journal your feelings and reflect on them (or try Noting).

Noting is the act of labelling the thoughts that go through our head. This does not only name what we are feeling and bring the emotion into view, but it also allows us to try to explain why we might feel like this. Using this technique can start the process of understanding our feelings and trying to identify possible causes for them. The aim of "noting" is to reduce the control of the thought or emotion on our minds and increase our objectivity about our experiences. Noting can be done whenever during the day but the effects are most visible when your mind is clear (e.g. meditations) and you have minimal distractions.

This is one Noting technique:
1. Sit somewhere comfortable and set a timer for 5 minutes (Longer than a minute will do).

2. As you become aware of the thoughts that pop into your mind begin to start writing or 'Noting' them down. Try using the form "I am thinking of X". E.g. "I am thinking about work.", "I am thinking about tomorrow", "I am thinking about my thinking.". Stop after your timer finishes.

3. Now describe your thoughts as objectively as possible, without analysing or judging your experiences. Try not to use this format "I don't want to go to work. This day is going to suck!". Try to use this instead try this "I acknowledge I feel anxious about the workload I currently have".

This technique can help us see the thoughts we are having through an objective lens and minimise our reaction to them. Being more aware of the flow of our own thoughts can help normalise our mental processes. However, if your negative moods persist or you are finding them too difficult, please contact your GP or mental health professional. There are other ways to access formal help listed in the "If you need some extra help section".

Friends, Family and Others

Disclosing how we are feeling to a family member, friend or another person can be equally helpful.

If there isn't a person that you feel comfortable speaking to that's okay! There are plenty of free support services active in the UK with support workers at the end of the phone waiting for you to call. You don't need to be in a crisis to access them!

If there are people you feel comfortable speaking to that is equally as helpful. One way to start is to create a list of people whom you would consider talking to. Think of what the pros and cons are for speaking with each person as well as, the pros and cons of not speaking with them (this is important too). If you feel unsure whether you want to speak to someone, watch how they receive different types of news. This can be a great way of determining how they receive information and if they're the right person for you to talk to.

Once you have chosen someone, pick a time that they are free. Plan what you're going to say and how you're going to say it. You can start with thinking of examples about what you want to speak about and work backwards to think what you want to talk to them about. Try to be honest about what you want to speak about and use examples if that helps. Remember that you don't need to share everything all at once! Another good area to touch on is how you want to be supported now and in the future.

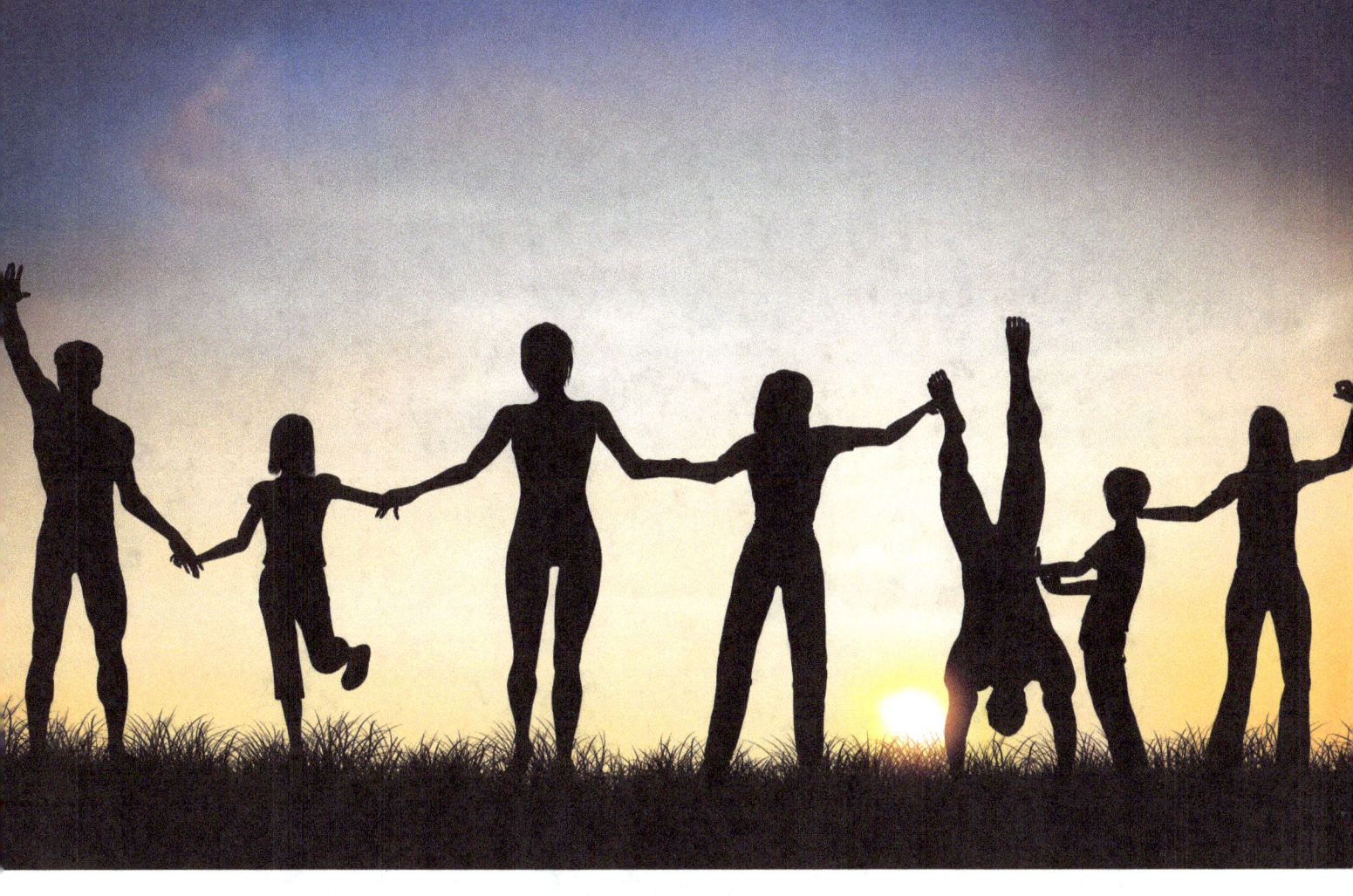

Sometimes the recipient won't know the right thing to say and may react in a way that you didn't expect at first. This is okay, allow them to take time and think about what you have told them. Then if possible, plan to return to the conversation at a later date to try again. If they don't react in the right way and continue to do so, try talking with someone else about their reaction. You can talk with someone whom you have previously spoken to, your GP, a medical and mental health professional, or a superior in your job.

Creating a relationship with someone, yourself included, can be an enriching and positive experience for your own wellbeing.

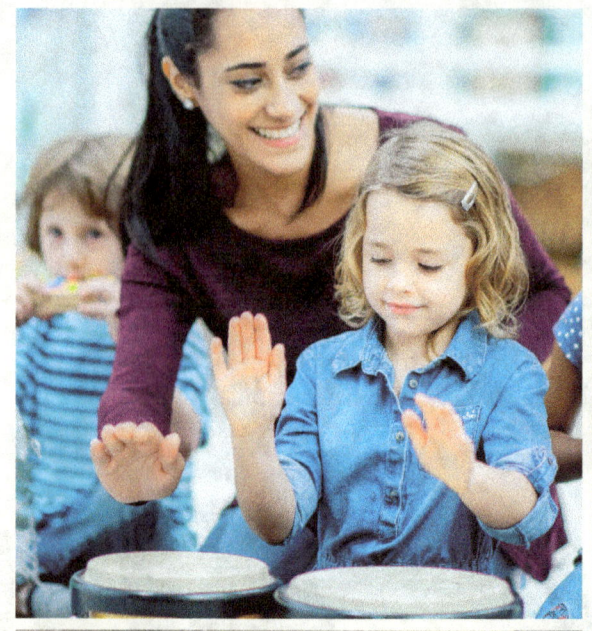
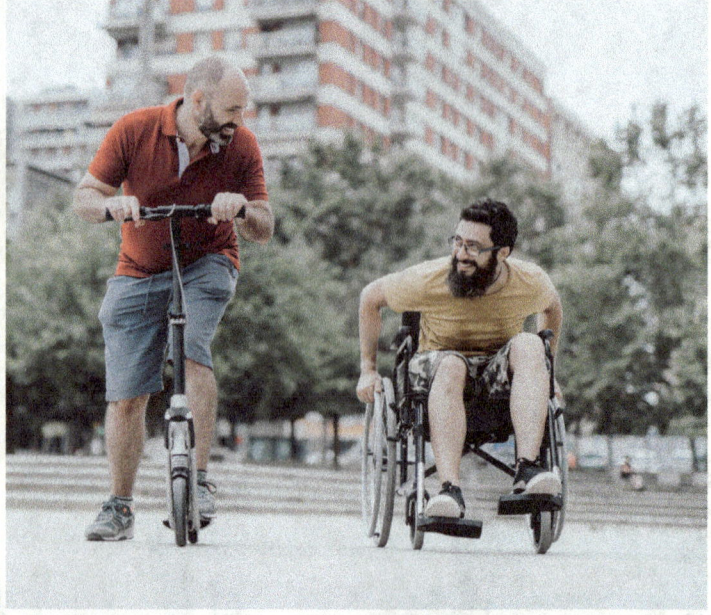
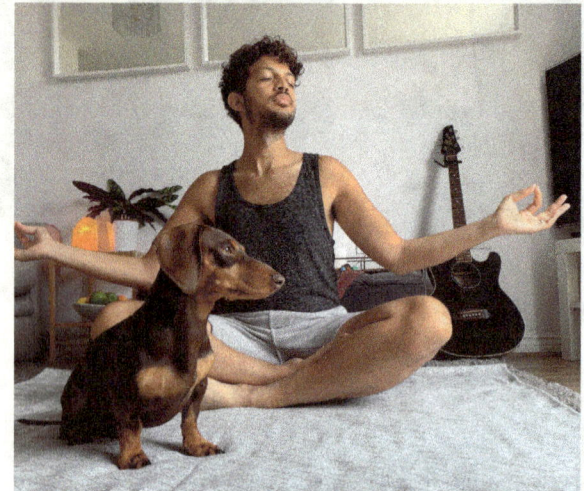

MANY WAYS TO MEDITATION

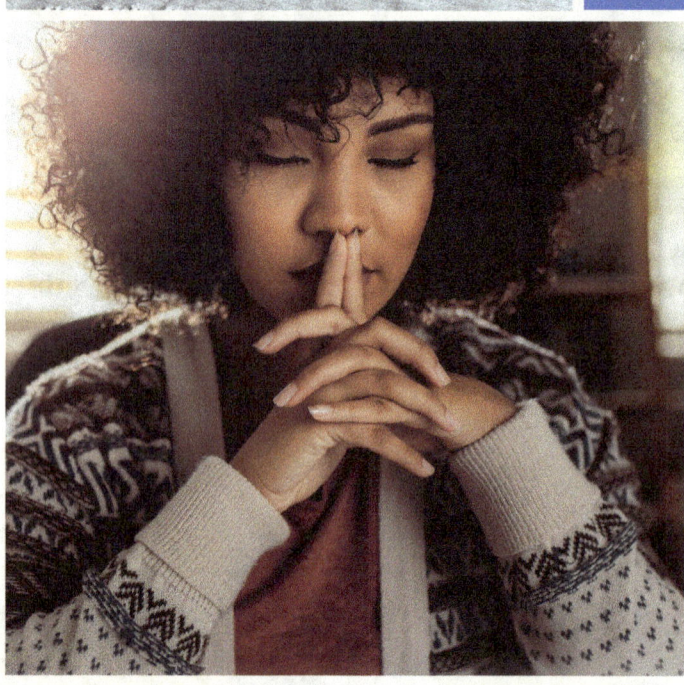
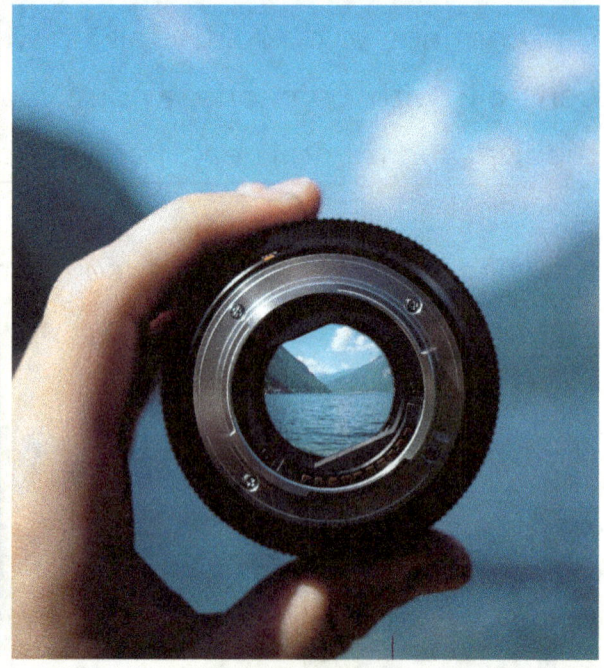

Meditation

Meditation is about training our minds to view the world from a healthy state of awareness without self-judgement. This doesn't specifically refer to the act of someone sitting cross-legged on the floor for hours at a time. That is a type of meditation, but meditation is a skill that can be used in many areas of our lives. Meditation helps us foster an awareness of the world by training our mind to live with full attention and be present.

This is why many activities count as meditation like: playing a musical instrument, looking at art, focusing on our breath and almost everything else you can think of. There are plenty of fantastic physiological and psychological reasons to meditate like: reducing stress hormones and healing times as well as increasing our memory, creativity and creating compassion. Try some of these practices to begin your meditation journey -

CLARITY MEDITATION

1. Pick 2 colours, imagine one entering your lungs and filling them up and then a 'dirty colour' exiting your lungs

2. Go through your body top to bottom and feel how each muscle is – tense/relaxed

3. Before sleeping repeat the same as 2. but while relaxing

4. Go through your body and feel what is in contact with it, the feeling of the weight of your body (feet, arms, bottom) on the surface

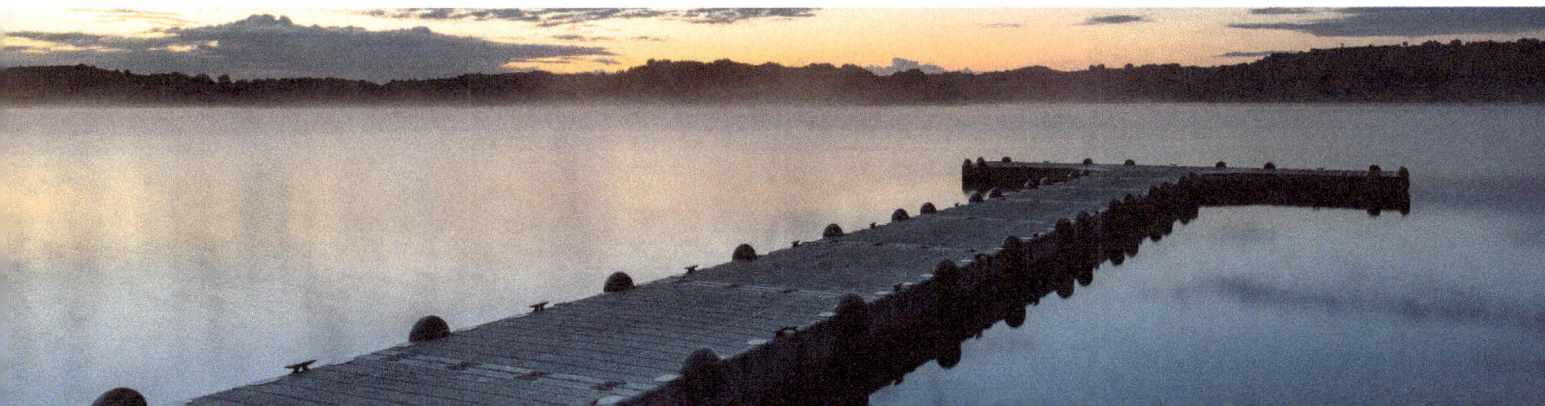

Meditation of relaxation

Relaxation is important especially when our lives are so busy but when was the last time you focused on relaxation? Giving yourself the time to relax and unwind from the day's events is an extremely important element to keep yourself well. The goal of "Relaxation Meditation" is to clear your mind and allow yourself to relax. You can practice this method anywhere but try to be somewhere quiet and comfortable. You can complete this standing up or even lie down but for the best results try sitting upright on something with a hardback and with your feet on the ground. Raise your body up straight, roll your shoulders back and place your hands flat on your legs (or surface). Have your gaze (eyes open or closed) about 45 degrees downward. Relax into your comfortable position and begin...

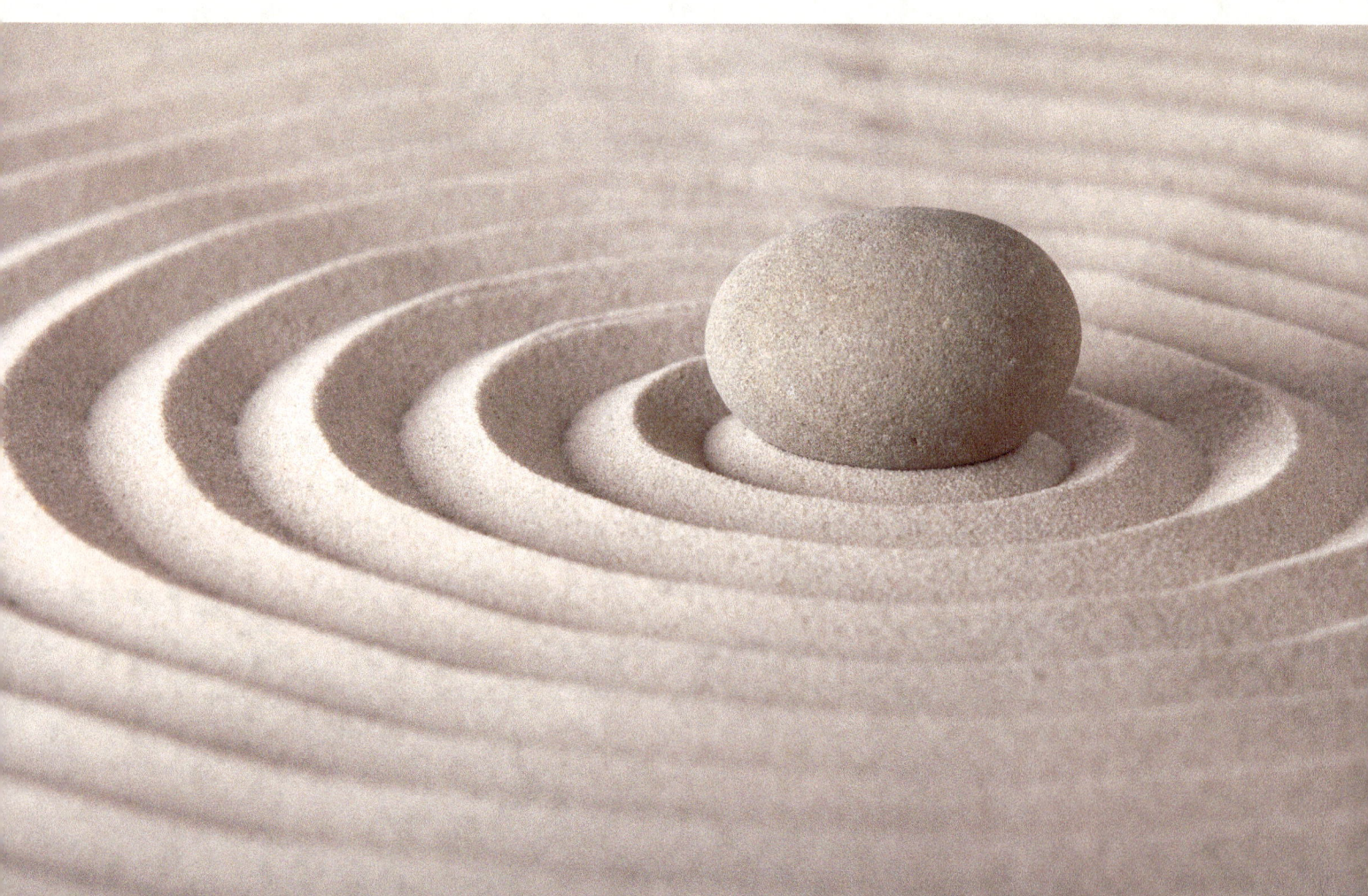

1. Breathe deeply and focus on your breath - Start by taking three to five deep breaths with eyes closed in a seated posture. This can be any way you like but breathing in through the nose and out through the mouth works best for some. Focus on the air you're inhaling. Focusing on every part of your body where you can feel the breath. Noticing the subtle feelings throughout the journey of the breath. Imagine that when you exhale your breath all of the stress in your mind and body releases.

2. Body scan - Begin to breathe as you otherwise would, maintaining your awareness of the breath. Now start observing your body from head to toe, noticing any tension or discomfort. Scan a second time, observing which parts of the body feel a certain emotion. Take as long as you like but try to complete 3 scans in the time you have given yourself.

3. Awareness and breath - Notice any thoughts that arise without trying to label or change them. Note your mood and unjudgementally sit with the way you are feeling. Now return to your breathing, noticing the sensations once again. Count the breaths in your head from 1 to 10. Count at the end of the inhale or exhale. Once you have counted to 10 starts again at 1. If thoughts begin to enter your mind or your concentration starts to wander, don't worry. Just guide your attention back to the breath. Try doing this for five minutes or more if you like.

4. Finishing - Once you are ready to finish open your eyes and remain sitting for 20 seconds. Allow your mind to remain in a meditative state. It doesn't matter whether you're calm and focused or irritated by thoughts. Allow your mind to simply be. To finish your practice bring yourself back to your senses. What can you feel, see, taste, hear, smell? Remain aware and relaxed and continue with your day.

Mindfulness

Mindfulness is very closely linked to meditation, but it deserves its own section! Mindfulness is the human ability to be present in the moment, be aware of your surroundings and what you are doing. It helps us not become overwhelmed by what is going on around us or in our own heads. There are lots of different ways to remain present throughout your day and here are a few.

HOW TO PRACTICE MINDFULNESS:

1. Time - Set aside some time and find a space that you find comfortable

2. The present - Pay attention to the present moment as it is, without judgement

3. Mental note – When you notice a judgement such as a thought or feeling, make a mental note of them and let it pass

4. Return to the present – We often get carried away in thought, so return to the present moment.

5. Do not judge yourself – Recognise when your mind has wandered off and don't judge yourself for the thoughts that come up in your mind.

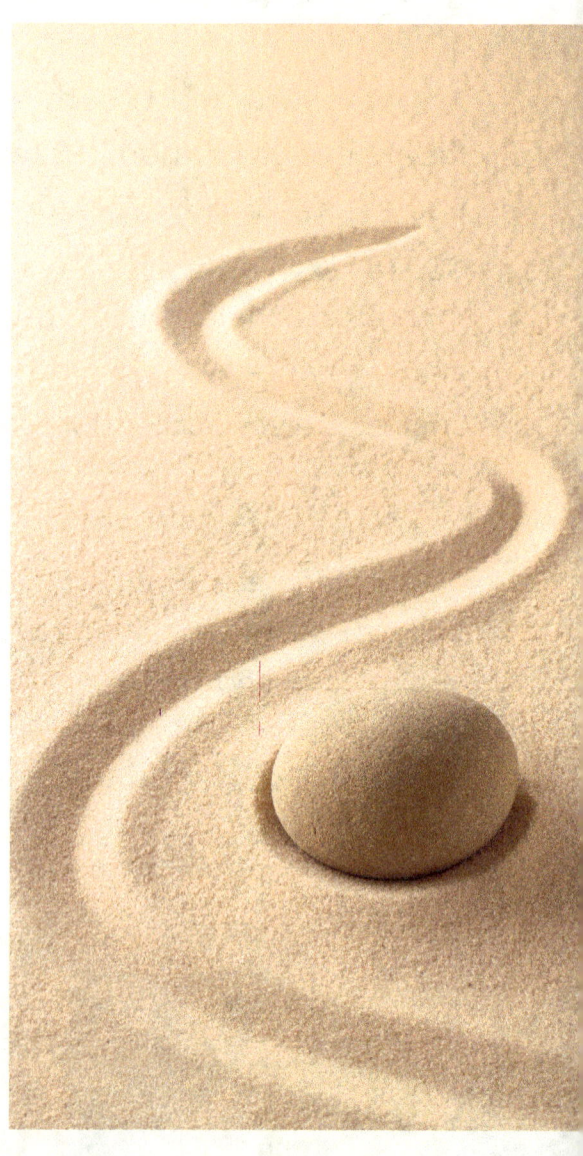

Mindful walk

1. Pick a regular walk you do everyday, roughly taking you 5 minutes. This can be anywhere you want to be as long as you can safely pay attention to your body at this time.

2. Begin by paying attention to your feet. Think about the sensations you're feeling on the soles of your feet. How each toe makes contact with the ground. The weight on each part of your foot.

3. Then begin to take notice of your other senses one at a time. Look up at the top of the buildings or notice a green tree. Feel the air on your face or the feel of your jumper. Notice the sounds of the road. Smell the aroma of that new restaurant.

4. Focus on one of each of these at a time. Try to ground yourself in the moment you're currently experiencing. When you're approaching the end of your walk return to your feet before you finish your walk. Equally you can use other techniques in this booklet to end your Mind Walk e.g. use your daily affirmation (pp.X) or view your thoughts from an external point of view (pp.X).

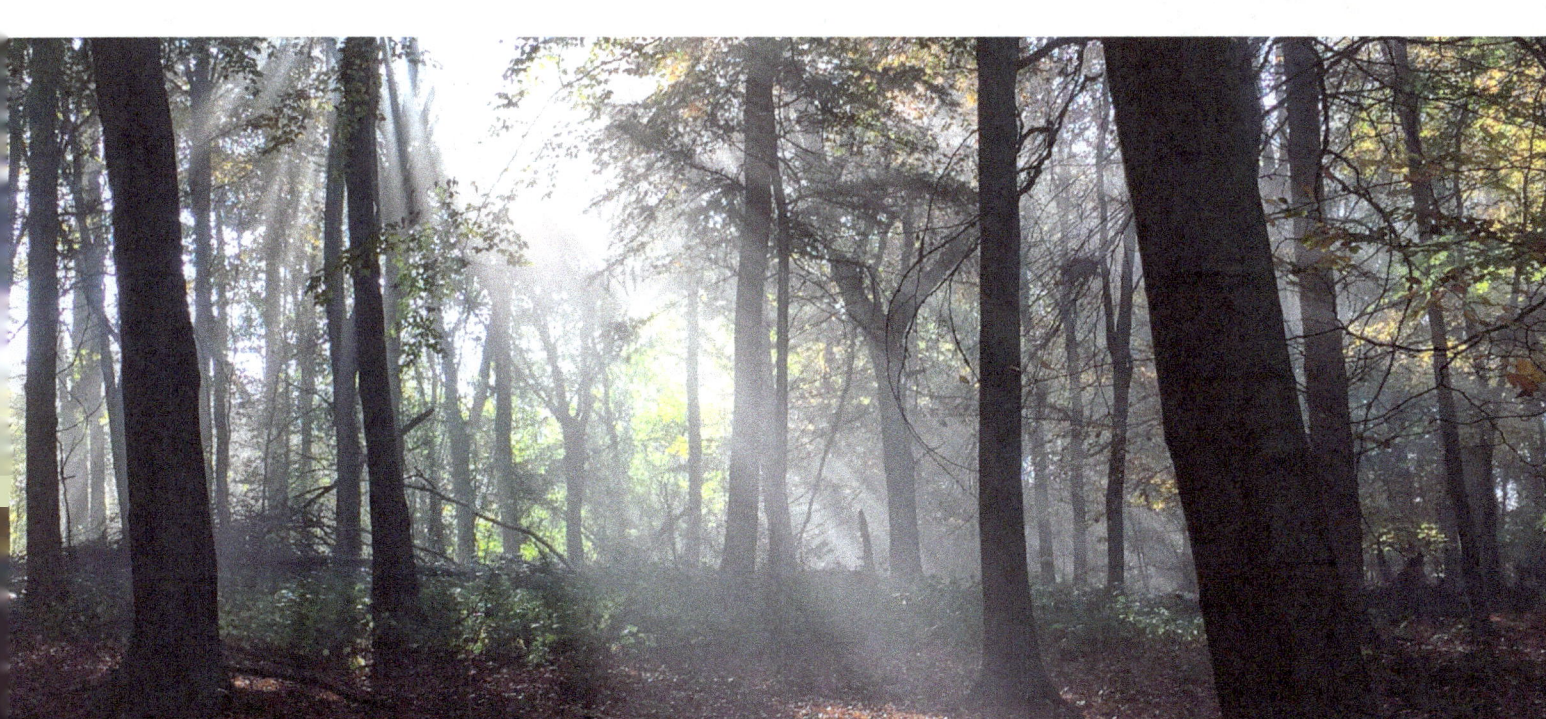

Mindful Eating

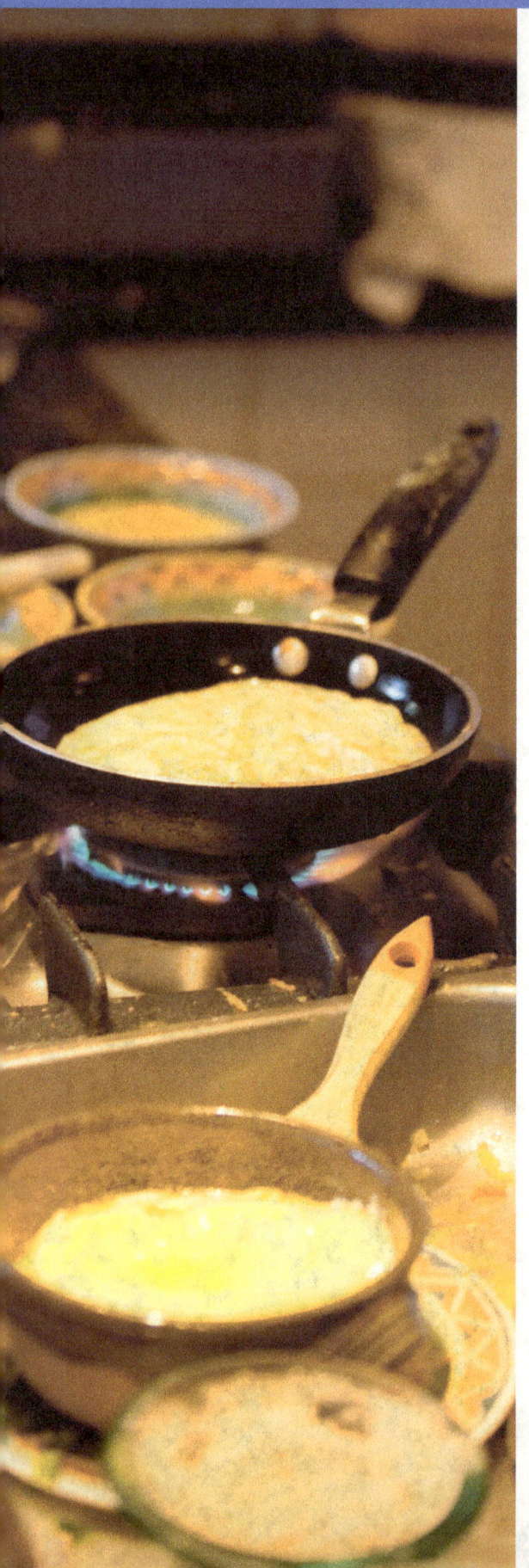

1. Look at the food you're about to eat. Take in how it smells, what size, shape and colour it is, what your feelings are towards eating this mouthful.

2. Take a bite and then put your cutlery down - What flavours do you taste? How does it feel in your mouth? What is the food's texture? Try to identify the flavours you're experiencing and how each of them feel.

3. Swallow and focus on the physical sensations throughout your body. How does it feel in your stomach? Contemplate the taste in your mouth. Try to see what flavour remains after you swallow. Think about the enjoyment of that mouthful.

4. Try to reflect a moment before continuing with your next mouthful. Did you enjoy the sensations? Do you want more or do you feel full? What is the current sensation in your stomach? Then continue the process again.

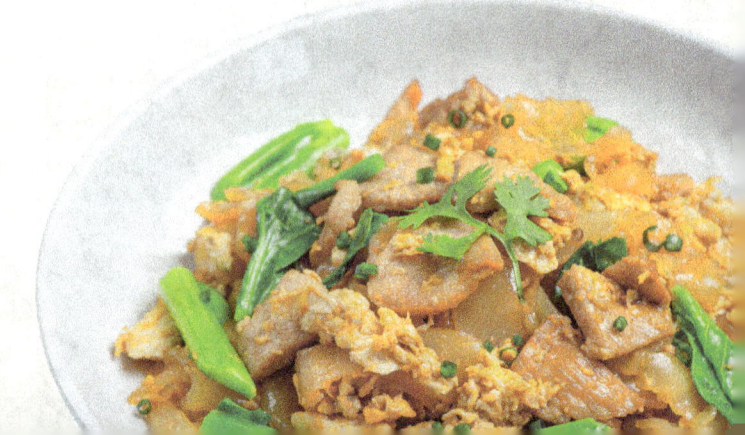

Mindful listening

1. Feelings – Ask yourself 'How am I feeling now?' Is there something getting in the way of being present for the other person? Do you need to address this now or can it wait till a later time?

2. Being present – Listen to the other person with interest, empathy and be open.

3. Reactions – Silently note your reactions – thoughts and feelings and return you attention to the other person.

4. Reflect – Paraphrase or summarise the main points of what the other person is saying, Make them feel heard

5. Acknowledge – Respect the other person's opinions; you do not have to agree, but acknowledge them before you introduce your own opinions.

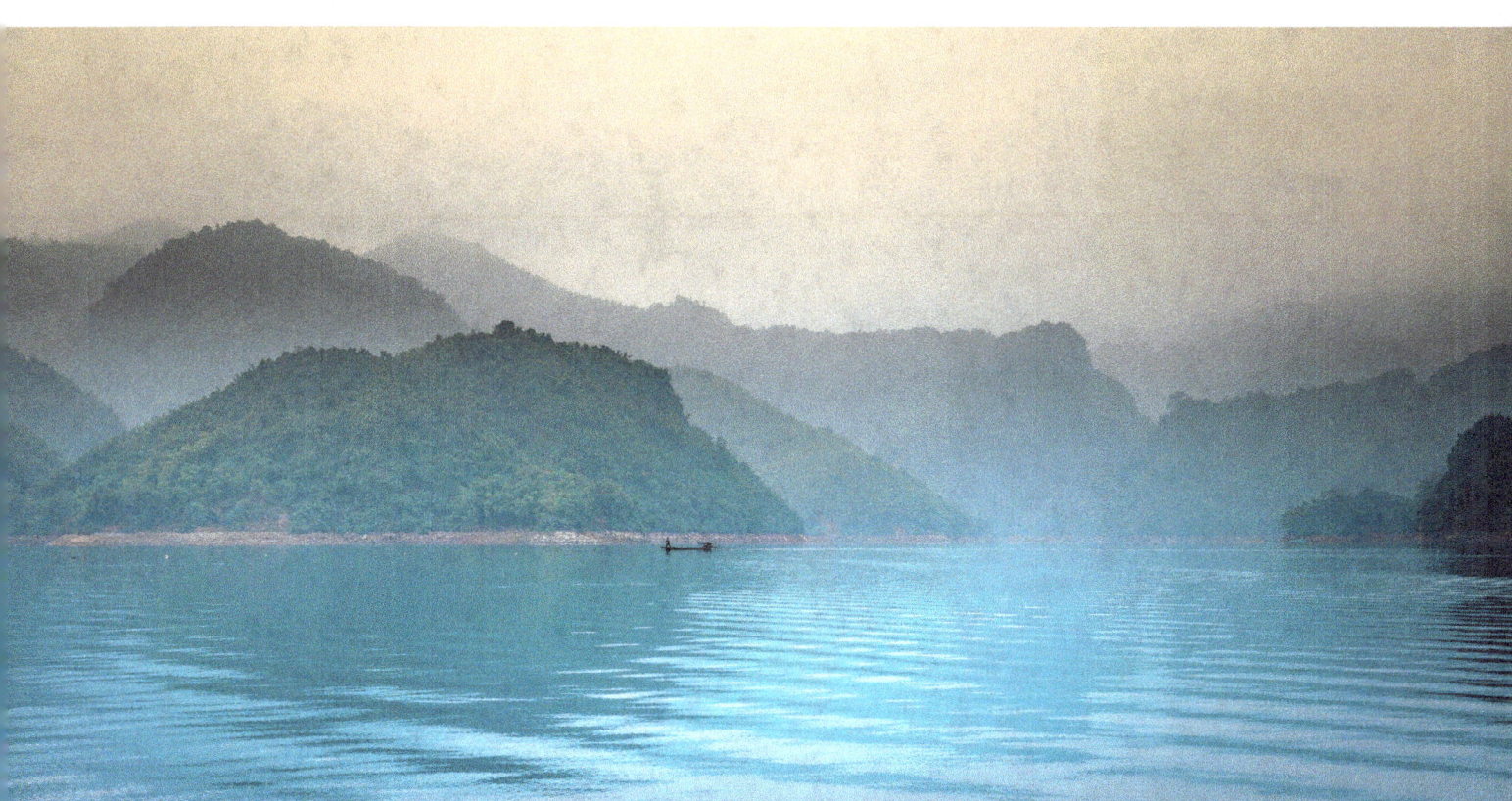

MAKING YOUR MOTTO

This personalised saying is a set of memorized phrases that are repeated silently whenever you want to give yourself compassion. The goal of this is to combat negative emotions when they arise by reminding you that you deserve kindness and happiness. Your saying will consist of three to four sentences that each invoke a feeling of positivity, strength and shared humanity.

1. The first sentence should try to label or acknowledge your experience objectively. Try some of the previous exercises in this booklet to understand your emotions before trying this. Examples - "I am not having a good time at this moment", "I am really suffering right now", "I am currently feeling unhappy and hopeless".

2. Your second sentence could remind you that suffering is a shared experience, and the feeling is impertinent. Try something like "I am not alone in suffering", "Others have got through this emotion, so I can too", "This is a shared experience by all", "Suffering is a part of life".

3. The third sentence should aim to bring caring concern for yourself in this moment. Try to think of something that might personally soothe you in that moment. E.g., "I can do this right now.", "I deserve love and affection", "May I give myself the kindness I need right now".

4. The last sentence is there to set your intention to be kind and considerate to yourself. For example - "I am enough. I do not need validation", "I will give myself the care I deserve", "I am worthy of happiness".

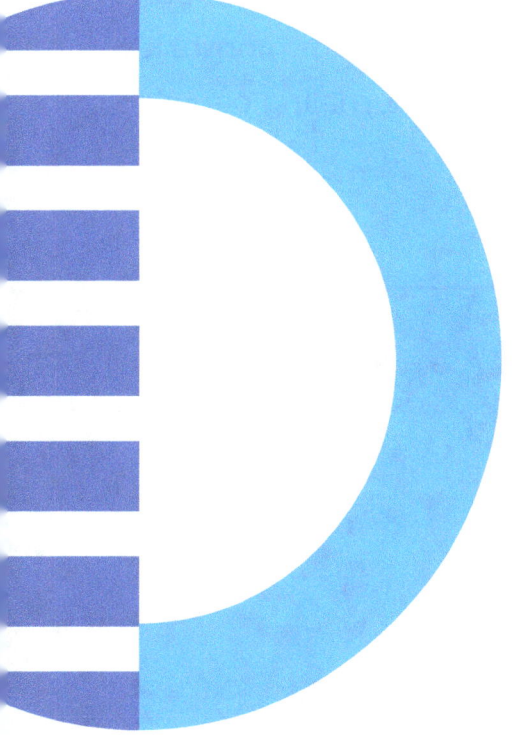

Once you have created your own personal MOTTO memorise it so you are ready for when you need it. Play around with where you put the emphasis in each sentence. This can help bring new life to your MOTTO when you have used it a lot. Try repeating it next time you need to look after yourself. It's a great and easy way to foster a positive outlook when things are difficult.

Journal writing

The best way to think of journaling is to think of it as simply just having a conversation with yourself. Ask yourself how you are feeling, and then respond to that feeling. Once you've written out your response, ask yourself what happened during the day that might've contributed to that feeling. More often than not, you'll find the answer that you're looking for.

For example - "I've not been feeling so great today, I've found myself quite on edge and anxious all day" Why do you feel like that, what happened? "Well, I probably had one too many coffees, but I've also not done any exercise in a few days."

By journaling, it allows you to get your thoughts and emotions out of your head and onto the paper. In there, we can find out the root of the problem and look at sorting it out. Journaling allows us to process our thoughts. Research has proven how good it is for both our mental and physical health. Give it a go!

Sound interesting? Now grab a pen and a book and get started! You can start whenever, it doesn't necessarily have to be at the start of a year or month. It's all about the present. If you're not a fan of writing by hand, journaling can also be done digitally. Try some of our examples out!

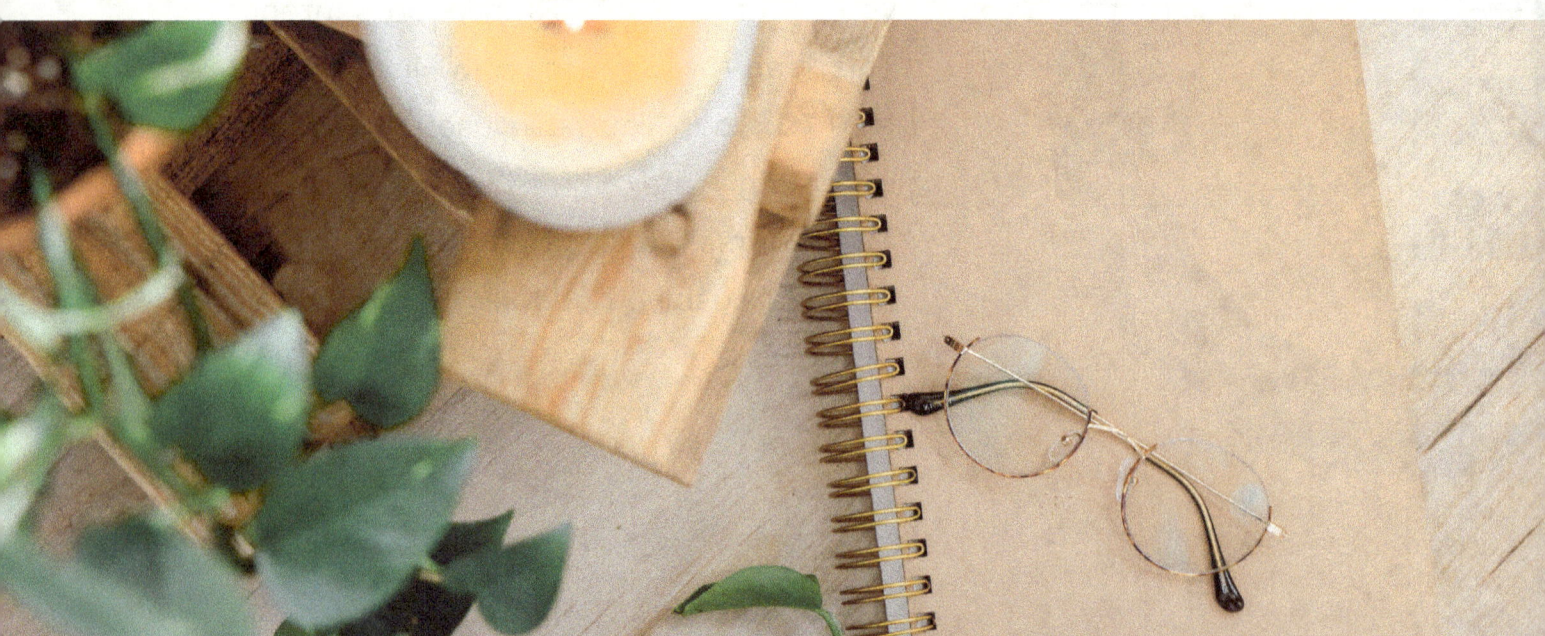

JOURNAL WRITING

The best things that happened today...

Things I wish I can change about today...

I am proud of myself today because...

I think I still need to work on...

Bullet Journaling

When it comes to journals and journal writing, we may think they are only used for writing about tasks that need to get done and important dates. Similarly, when we think of diaries, we think of wordy paragraphs about our feelings. What about those who want a flexible journal for both? Bullet journaling might be for you!

Bullet journaling is a planner system made to boost productivity. It can help with day-to-day organisation, but it can also be used to express emotions as well as aid us in our mindful and therapeutic techniques.

Dealing with first page fear

Toxic perfectionism – do not put pressure on yourself to make the first page look amazing, journaling is for you, and only for you to see.

Journals gets better over time and it gradually becomes an easier task to do – getting started is the hardest part.

Try experimenting and changing the format up – it will make things more interesting and give you more motivation to carry on.

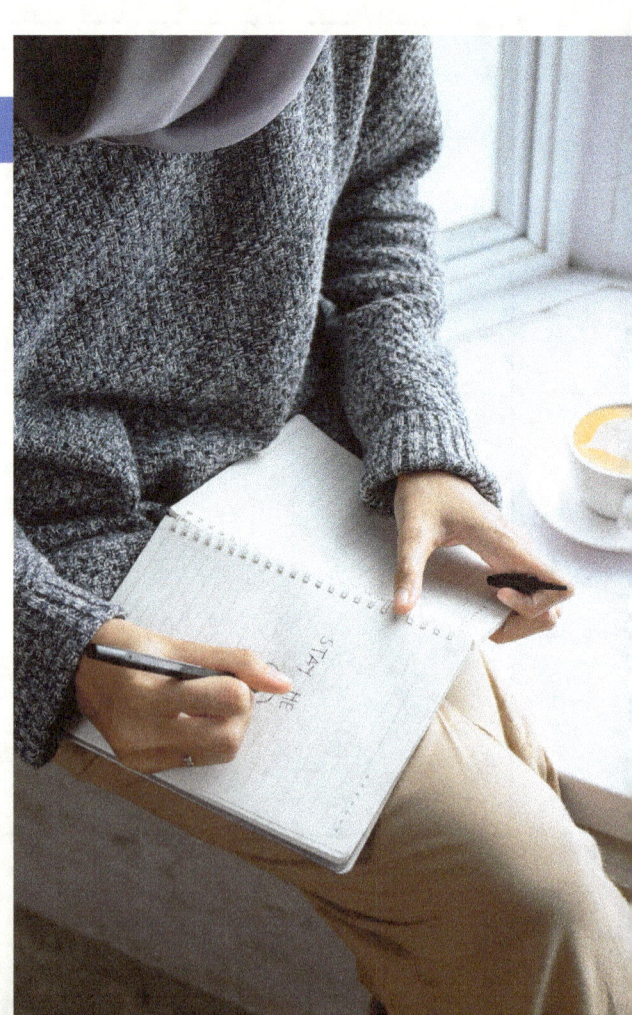

77

REFLECTION NOT RUMINATION

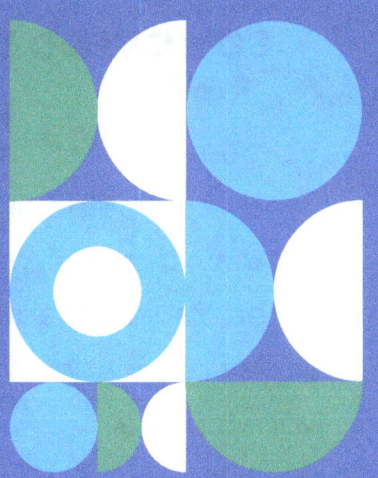

If you find yourself rethinking over an event or what someone else has said or done even if it was long ago, this is known as rumination. Rumination is a natural response to a problematic situation which can result in negative cycles that have the capacity to hinder mental health. When we choose to focus on memories of a loved one to keep them close to us this can be comforting for it serves a purpose. However, when we start to repetitively replay it over and over again this can associate with negative emotions and cause distress which is unhealthy for us. If your negative moods or thoughts persist or you are finding them too difficult please contact your family doctor or mental health professional. There are other ways to access formal help listed in the "If you need some extra help section" near the end of the book.

SO HOW DO YOU GO ABOUT STOPPING RUMINATION?

Set time aside each day to allow yourself to go over anything that may have caused you trouble or is worrying you. Try and not let it negatively impact your whole day, instead set 20 minutes aside in the evening to allow yourself to go over the issue. Scheduling in time to go over an issue can help keep the rest of your day rumination free whilst still allowing yourself time to think about what is worrying you.

Journal what went on and how you felt. Keeping a journal allows you to create a space where you can reflect on your experiences and discuss healthy coping strategies that you have tried or want to try. People tend to have a theme to their rumination, so it is helpful to recognise this and acknowledge how and why it is making you feel a certain way. This is a great step towards combatting the issue or thought.

When you notice the patterns often associated with rumination, distract yourself instead – move your body, count down from 5 and take deep breaths to take your mind elsewhere. You can do this through meditation or mindfulness, or just focus on what you need to do in your day. Some thoughts are best left, so that you can focus on the more positive ones.

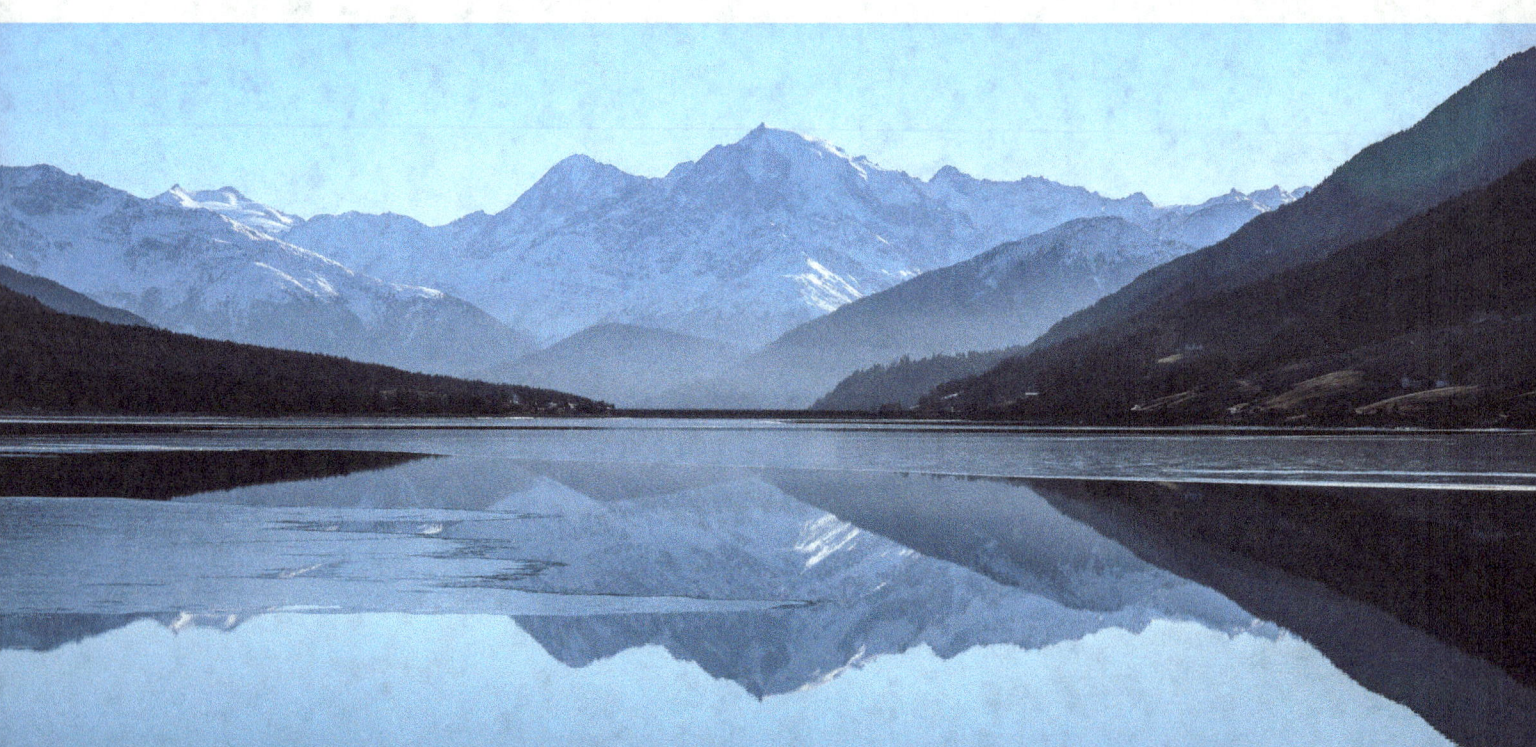

The difference being that reflection has intent for beneficial outcomes, it is a growth mindset that we can use to help improve our lives- it is similar to rumination in the sense that we focus on our past experiences without the negativity attached. Reflection allows us to learn through experience and focus on the positive aspects that went well, this can be tricky for most of us hence why rumination comes into play. Reflection allows you to take control over your feelings and behaviours and come to terms with why and how to improve going forward or perhaps reveal something about yourself. A beneficial aspect of reflection is that it influences self-confidence as you acknowledge yourself and what motivates you to be the best you. If you are always stuck in the past you may end up creating patterns of rumination. To help move forward and achieve, it is important to reflect not ruminate. Reflecting on our thoughts and experiences and learning from them helps us grow as humans. We can use our experiences constructively and without pain. Turning your rumination into healthy reflection can help improve your wellbeing and mental health.

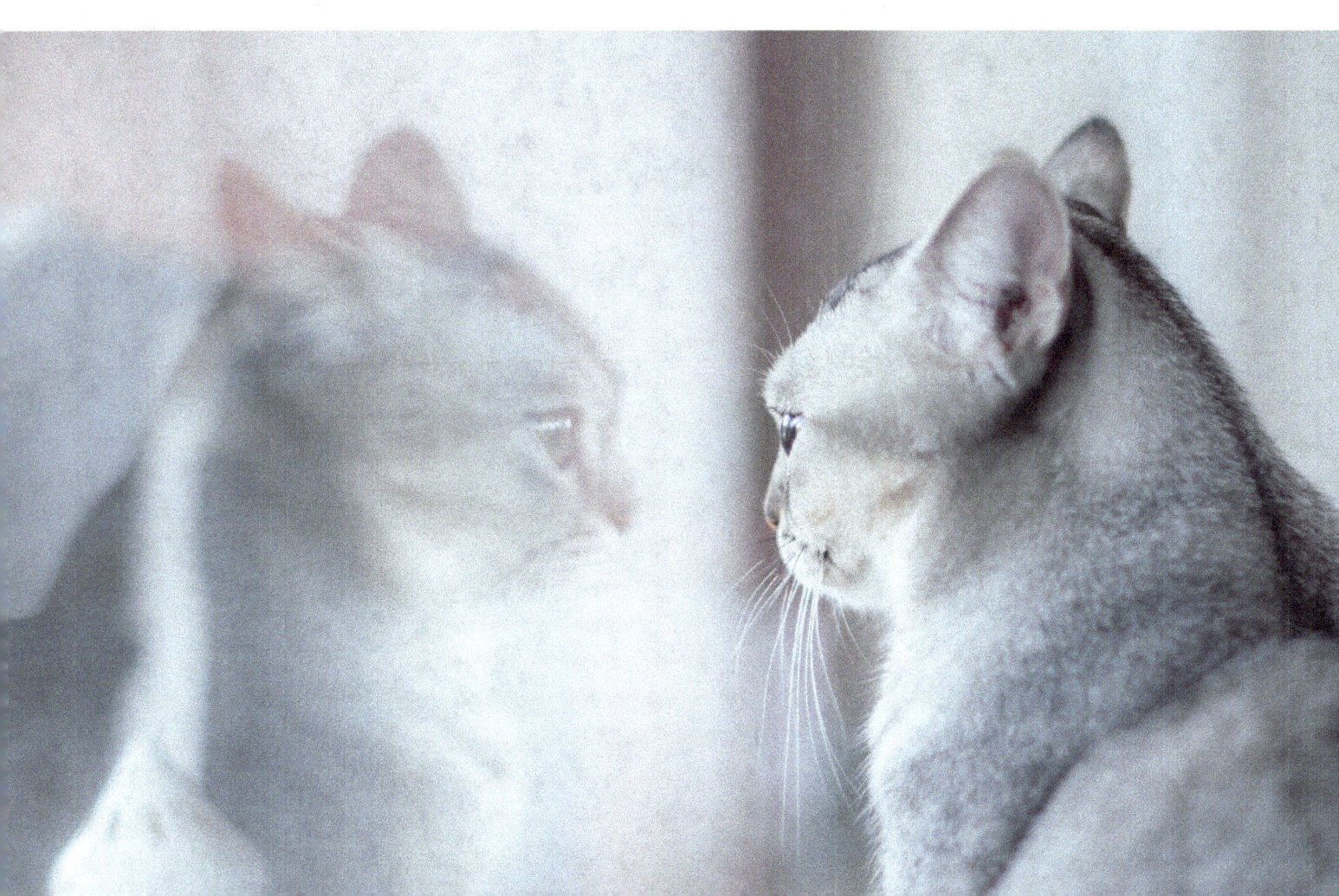

4

If you're not feeling too great

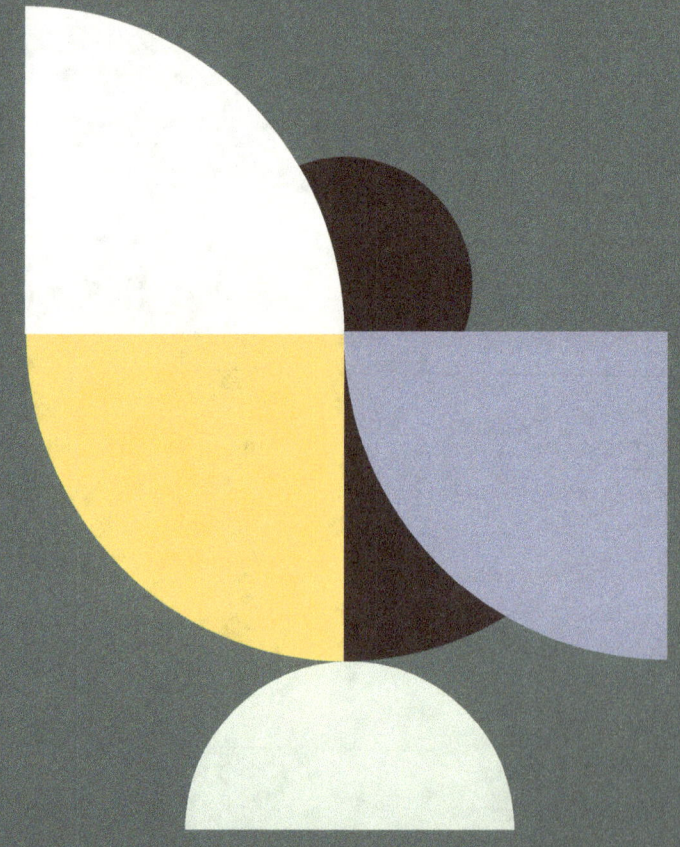

If you're not feeling too great

This section is for when things haven't been going well for you and you want to try and change that. It is normal to have fluctuations in our mood but if this experience is prolonged and/or severely affecting us we should always reach out for additional help. You can find a guide to this in the section "If you're not feeling too great" however, always contact a medical or psychological professional if you're in doubt of where to go. This is a guide for advice only, and is not a substitute for professional help. However, this section aims to help you if you are not in a good place and want to try some self-help.

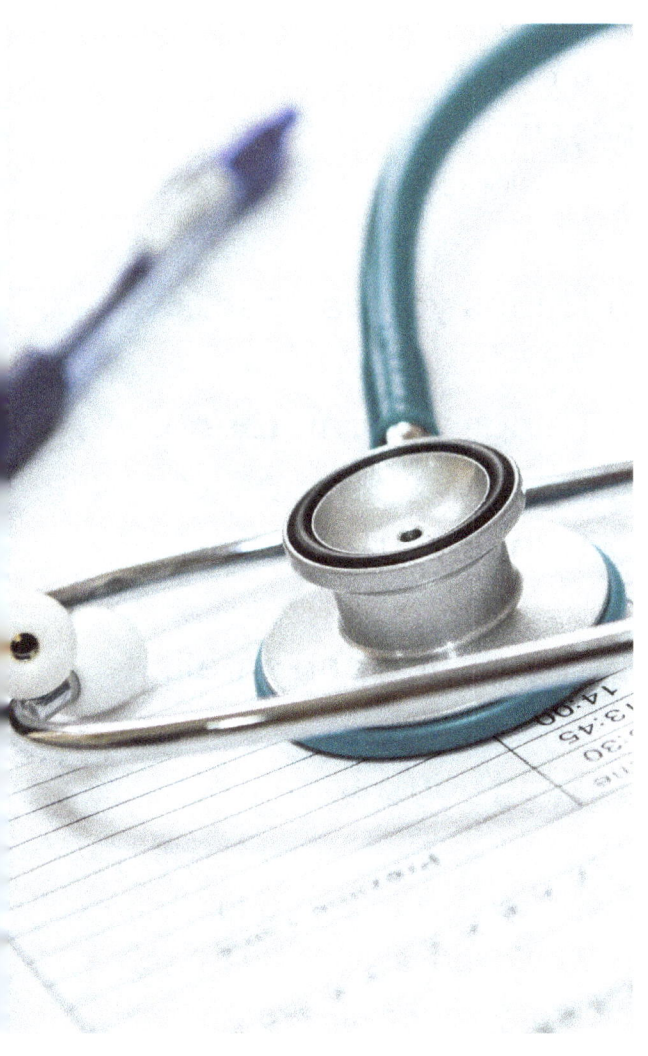
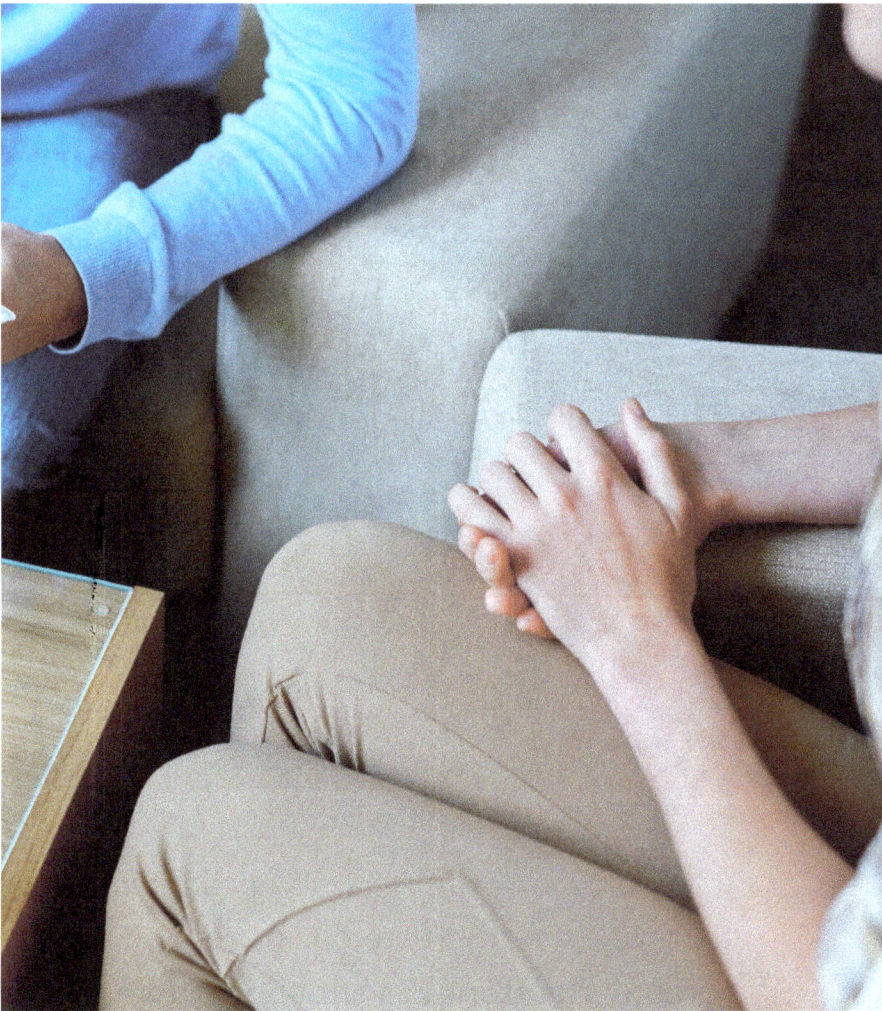

Grounding

Most people will have experienced the emotion of anxiety at least once within their lifetime. For some people it will have a greater impact on their daily life than others. Often with anxious feelings you will begin to feel your senses overwhelming you and find it hard to keep track of your thoughts. We can sometimes enter a flight-or-fight response where our body produces stress hormones such as adrenaline and cortisol. This activates the autonomic system and causes physiological changes which can help us tackle the situation. However, this reaction can be inappropriate and leave us in a negative way. Using a technique such as the 5-4-3-2-1 grounding techniques can become useful in a situation like this by trying to 'ground' you and help you focus on your surroundings in order to calm the flurry of thoughts. This is just one way in which you may choose to ground yourself but there are other techniques so it's important that you find a way that works best for you.

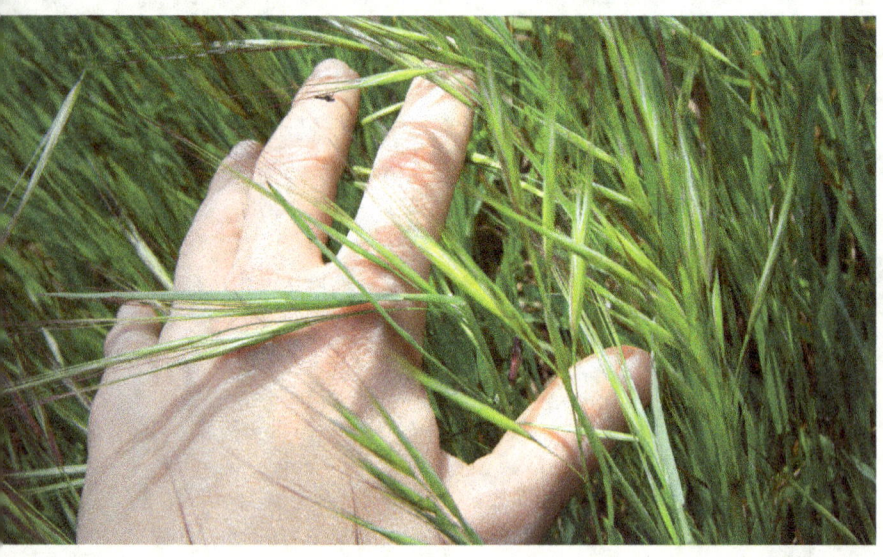

5 Things you can see.

4 Things you can touch.

3 Things you can hear.

2 Things you can smell.

1 Thing you can taste.

It may be helpful if this is a technique you use often, to talk through this technique with trusted friends or family who would be able to walk you through the steps in a situation where you yourself may not be able to.

Self Expression

Self-expression is a display of individuality whether it is through words, clothing, hairstyle, art, etc. Self-expression is an essential part of our lives; it allows us to experience something new or practice one of our passions. Self-expression involves any activity where we can transfer the energy from our thoughts and feelings into another form. When we express our feelings honestly, we are better equipped to deal with their repercussions because we have a greater understanding of what we are feeling.

Sometimes It can be tricky to start self-expression if you are not sure how to access creativity or inspiration. Here are a few ideas to practice self-expression:

Inner Child: Draw yourself as a child on a piece of paper. Add images and words to give this child everything that it needs, including a supportive nurturing parent.

Inside – Outside Bags/Boxes: Decorate a bag or box with images and words on the outside to represent the qualities you show to the world. Decorate the inside of the bag or box with images and words that represent the inner qualities that are hidden to most people.

Inspired Poem: Think of a quote that is meaningful to you and write it at the top of a piece of paper. Add your own lines below it that expand on the quote in the way you understand it – continue for the rest of the page. If you want you can find someone to read your poem for you while you use movement or gesture to express the meaning of your words.

Four Elements of You: Fold a piece of paper into four sections. Label each section, The Earth of Me, The Air of Me, The Fire of Me, and The Water of Me. Use images and colours to express your passions in life as symbolized by the four elements.

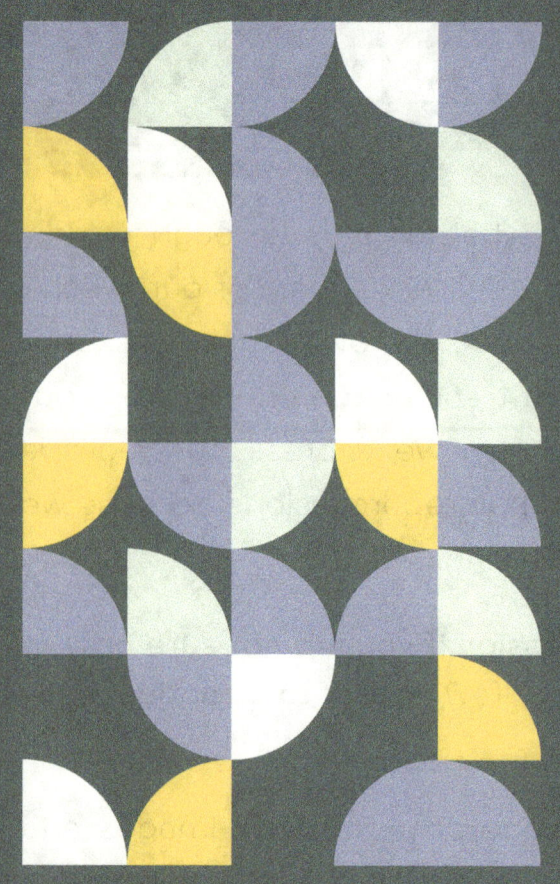

EXPRESS

YOURSELF

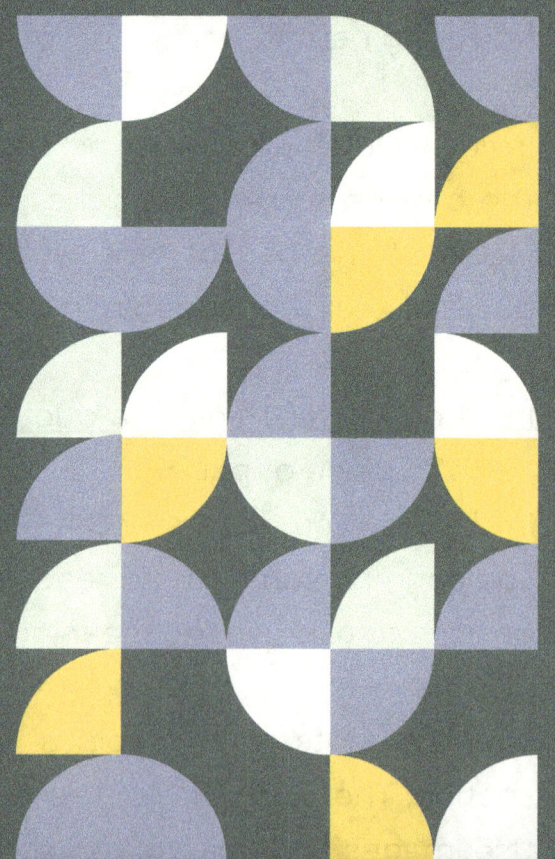

Hobbies

Another way to self-express is to find a hobby that you enjoy spending time on. Finding a new hobby or continuing with an old one can help you improve your mental health and wellbeing. Research has shown that people with hobbies are less likely to suffer from adverse mental health and poor wellbeing. Activities that get you out and about can make you feel happier and more relaxed. Here are a few tips:

Transform What You Already Enjoy Into a Hobby

Look at the ways you already enjoy spending your time and figure out how they can become hobbies. You are already doing things you love. The easiest way to find hobbies that you truly enjoy is to figure out how to build off those things.

Reclaim Your Childhood Interests

Think about the hobbies you used to enjoy before adulthood when you were a child, you probably had hobbies you loved, so revisiting them as an an adult can be a great way to find a hobby you enjoy.

Take an Assessment

There are several test and assessments online that are geared at finding a hobby that fits your personality traits. Have a look to see if you can find one.

Start Trying Things and See What Sticks

The truth is, no matter how you approach finding a new hobby, it can be hit or miss. The only way you can know for sure if you are going to like something is by giving it a go. It might take a few attempts to find a hobby that you love, but the key is to not give up. Eventually, you'll find a hobby that feels like the right fit for you.

There are no downsides to Self-Expression, only a multitude of benefits. Learning to understand yourself and more effectively express your thoughts and feelings is A great way for improving your mood, confidence and overall wellbeing.

SELF-CARE TRACKER

Choose a couple of self-care gestures that you want to ensure that you do. Use the tracker below to ensure that you are keeping on top of them over the next month. To use it every month - just use a pencil!

	Week 1	Week 2	Week 3	Week 4
Eg. Turn off screens at 10pm	✓			

 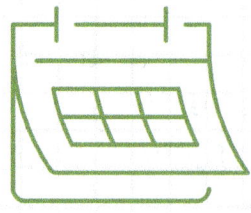  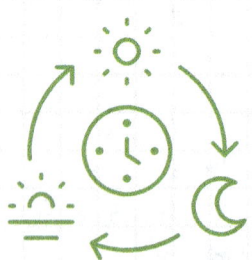

Thought Catching

It is normal to have negative thoughts from time to time. These thoughts can influence our moods, emotions, behaviours and physical reactions. If these thoughts keep reoccurring for a long period of time or are severely impacting your life, make sure you contact your GP or mental help professional – To note, thoughts of suicide are never normal and indicates that there is an underlying mood disorder that needs addressing - please see the "If you're not feeling too great" section towards the end of the book for more information. If these thoughts are not what has been mentioned you can try this technique. This technique aims to try and reduce how much these thoughts affect our lives and tries to change our mood for the better.

WHO ARE THEY?

Notice all your thoughts - Good, bad, and indifferent. Then work backwards and identify where the thought may have come from (you can use the other tools in this kit to help). Identifying the source can help us to face what is actually there.

Who are they coming from? Are these ultimatums made from yourself? Do your friends, co-workers and loved ones see you like this? Sometimes they can be predictions about yourself that have no backing. Check who and where these thoughts are coming from.

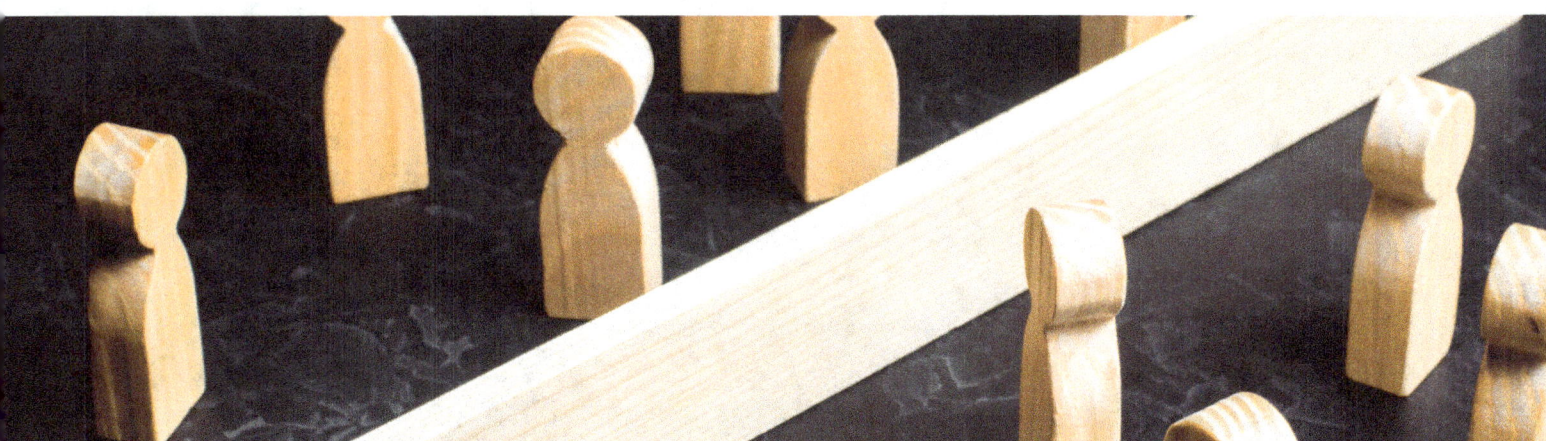

WHAT CAN WE DO?

Write down the answers to these 6 questions when a recurring thought enters your mind:

What situation did your thought come from?

What emotion was felt?

What was the thought and how much did you believe it?

What supporting evidence do you have for the thought?

What counter evidence do you have to go against the thought?

What alternative thought can you replace the old one with?

This method can try to help you understand where the thought comes from and how much it affects you. Try to look at this objectively like you have written about it and work out why this thought has come to you then.

Identifying can be a great first step towards changing how you feel. Try the NHS "Catch it App" or use the table below!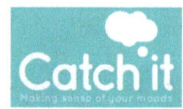

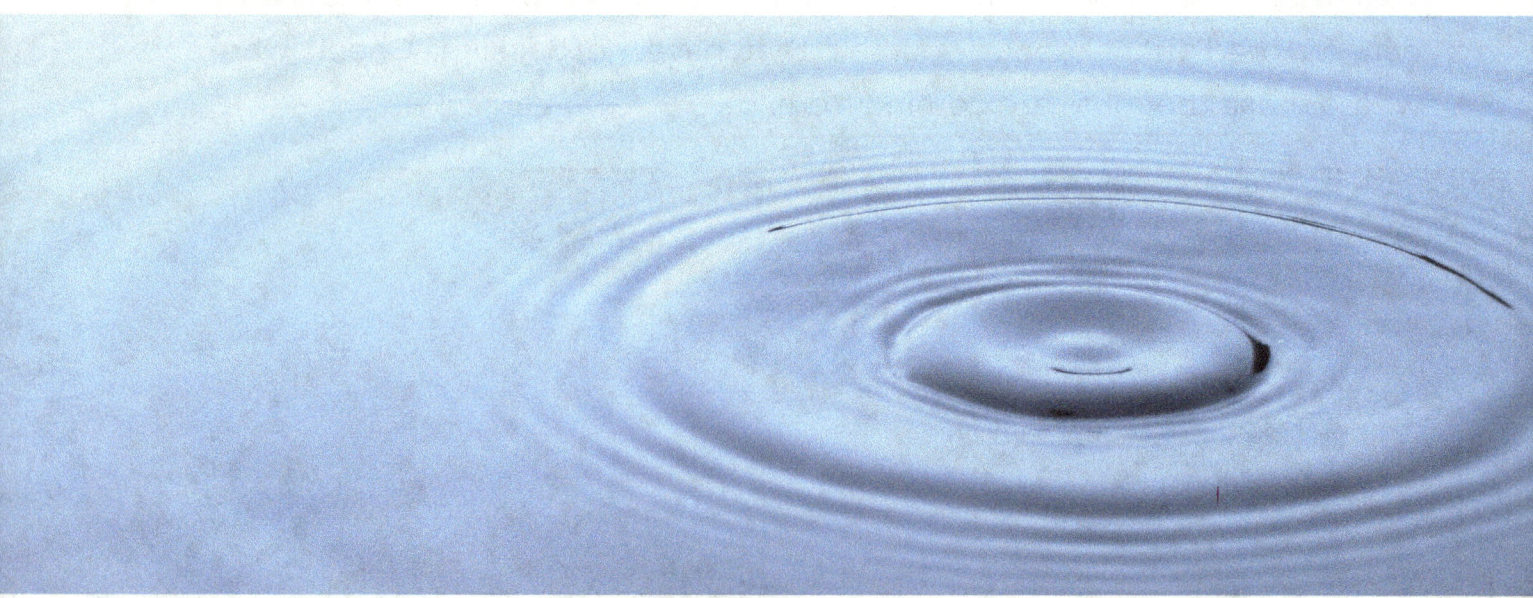

THOUGHT CATCHING

Situation	
Emotion	
Thought	
Supporting Evidence	
Counter Evidence	
Alternative Thought	

SITTING IN THE VALLEY

This last section can be very valuable in helping us understand our emotional states. This section is about staying with your negative emotion and trying to learn as much knowledge from it as possible. This process can help in improving moods faster, reduce stress levels and even improve physical health. However, if these thoughts keep reoccurring for a long period of time or are severely impacting your life make sure you contact your GP or mental health professional, please see "If you're not feeling too great" section towards the end of the book. For more information. This tool may not work or be appropriate for some individuals, do not feel pressured to have to do this one. We all work in our own unique ways. Beginning to move away from suppressing your emotions and moving towards an acceptance-based approach can feel like hard work at first but there are lots of reasons to stick at it.

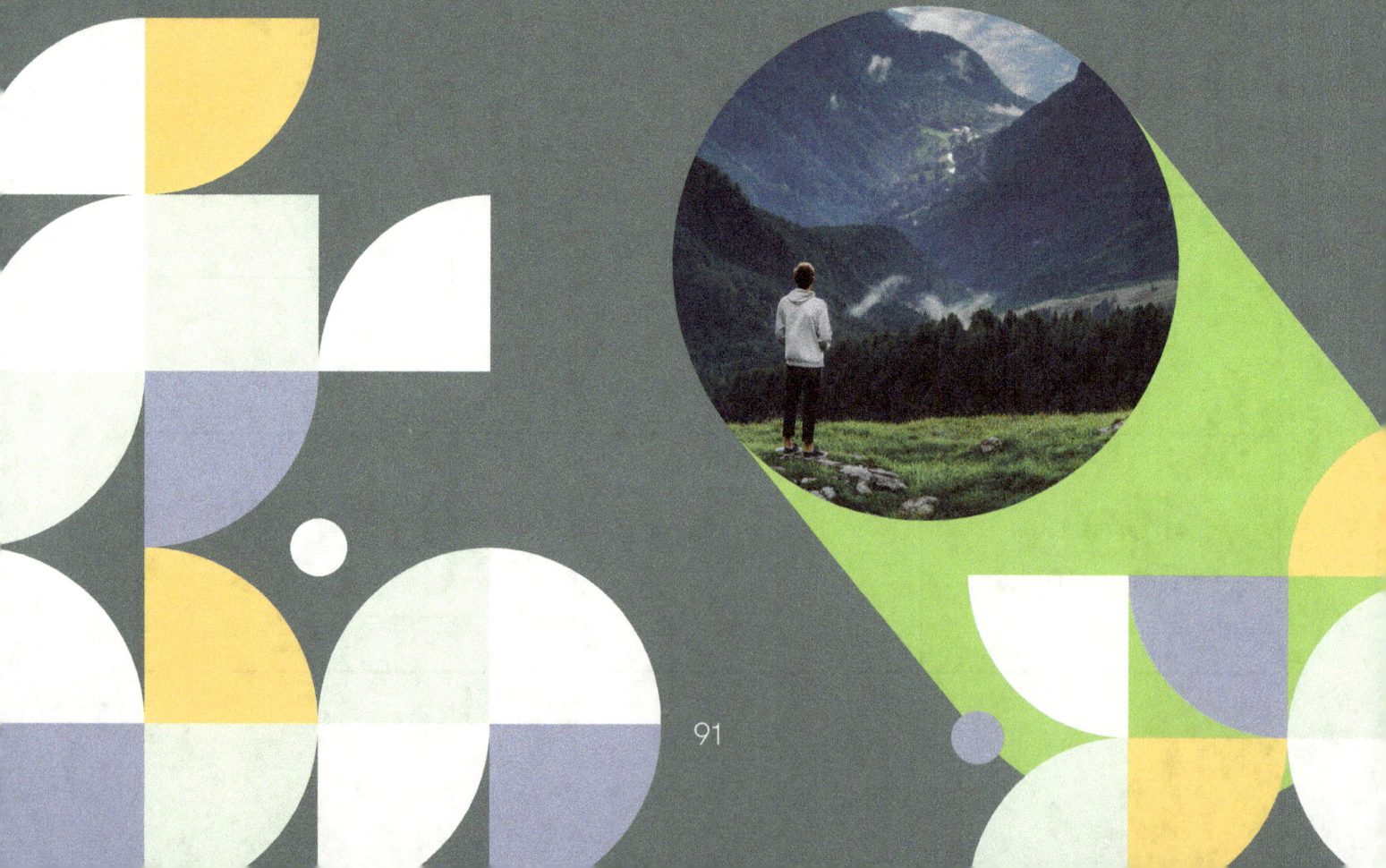

The avoided emotion will return either in the same state or within other situations, experiences or people. It can have the potential to propagate throughout a period of time and deny you control over your mind. Avoiding your emotions is avoiding your own mind. Your emotions are your own and although going through and living through negative emotions is not pleasant, it can be an enriching experience. Sometimes it tells you something important about your moods or gives you some insight into why you may be experiencing it. You can try sitting with your emotions by participating in this method:

1. Identify the emotion: Use the most prevalent emotion you are feeling. If you're experiencing more than one, come back and use the method with the next emotion.

2. Creating distance: Close your eyes and imagine picking the emotion out of you (where ever it feels like it comes from) and placing it 2 meters in front of you.

3. Creating form: Now create this emotion by answering the following questions. What size would this emotion be if it had to have one? What shape and colour would it be?

4. Reclaiming: Now watch the emotion you have created for a few moments and recognise what it is. Allow the emotion to return to where it came from inside of you.

5. Reflect: Reflect on what you have noticed about the experience. Notice what elements the emotion had. If this isn't the first time you've done this, how has the emotion changed? How did it feel? What was your reaction to it?

Try to practice this exercise as often as you can (preferably once a day or more). Look at the changes in how you represent the emotion and see how it evolves. See how you feel after giving your emotion form.

5

If you need a helping hand

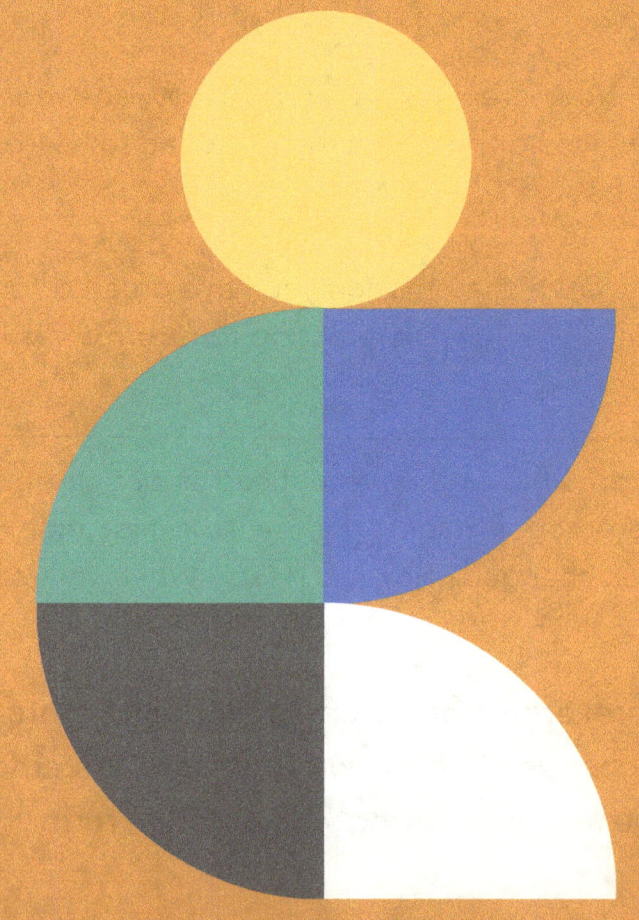

Talking With A Professional

Talking to someone about the negative issues that are going on in your life can help start the healing process. Sometimes your family and friends are not the right people you want to be listening to your worries, particularly if that problem concerns them. A professional mental health worker can provide us with an unbiased opinion and explore our concerns.

If you're experiencing symptoms such as weight loss, inability to concentrate, thoughts of suicide, struggles involving the consumption of food, excessive fluctuations in mood, intrusive thoughts, compulsions to perform certain activities, experiences of thoughts or sensual experiences not thought to be originating from oneself, please ensure you seek medical and psychological help.

Accessing professional help is a great positive step towards addressing whatever is going on. If you are having trouble with your mental health and/ or wellbeing there are trained individuals out there waiting to help. These are experienced professionals who are out there wanting to guide you towards better mental health.

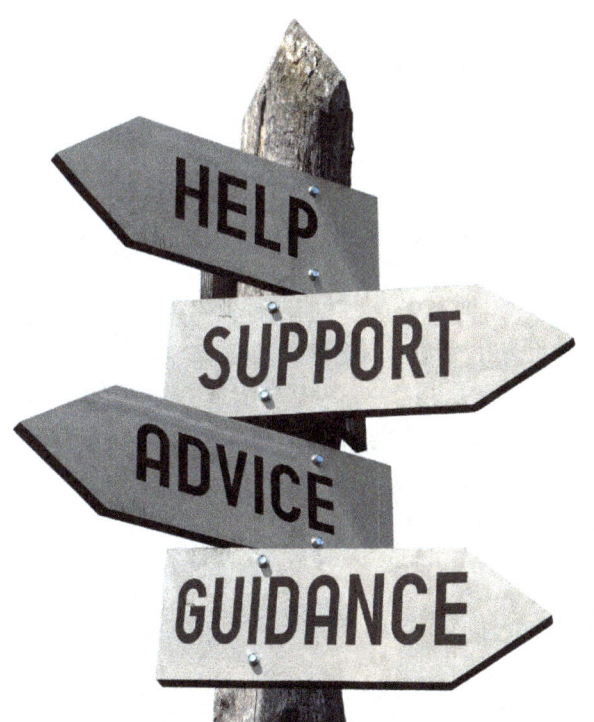

THE RE IS NO SHAME IN ASKING FOR HELP

94

Yourself

There are routes into counselling for free through the NHS in the UK. You can refer yourself or you can access this through a GP. For any type of counselling always ensure they are accredited with a professional body – BACP or UKCP. This tells you that they are acknowledged to have adequate levels of training and professionalism.

Your family doctor/general practitioner

Your family doctor can refer you to other professionals if you were comfortable with this. You can also choose to see a different GP if you don't feel comfortable speaking to your regular one.

Your superior

Most employers/institutes offer mental health resources or guidance. It is important that you inform someone (boss, HR, teacher, lecturer) in your workplace/place of study so that they are aware of how you are feeling. They will respect that it is not an easy thing to do but will help you get the right help and potentially provide additional measures to individually support you.

Counsellor

A counsellor is a professional aimed at providing non-judgemental support through whatever you are going through, They hope to provide a safe space where you both can explore possible avenues to help improve your mental health. Counselling can be accessible over the phone, in a group, via online chat services or in person.

It is important to remind yourself that there is no easy fix out there, just like a broken leg it takes time to heal and walk again. Mental health IMPROVEMENT is a work in progress, but it is worth investing your time in you.

Finding the right help online

The internet can be a great place to find support and there are so many options out there. Using online services can be great for finding information when you are going through a hard time. Finding out information about how you are feeling and wellbeing exercises you can do, can be a useful way to help make yourself feel empowered. However, other routes such as getting professional help can also be beneficial.

Finding information online and finding an online community can be great for educating yourself and seeking help. These sites provide an online space where you and different people can talk about experiences, symptoms, treatment and share support with each other. There are many different online communities, including professional and mental health specific communities and forums. Just remember that not all the information you find online will be reliable and trustworthy so keep that in mind. Sometimes it can feel like there is so much information out there, it can feel overwhelming, but finding correct and reliable information doesn't have to be.

HERE ARE SOME HELPFUL PLACES TO START:

Websites to find places to find information:
- The Be Free Campaign website
  www.befreecampaign.org
- NHS
- Mind – a mental health charity
- Mental Health foundation
- Rethink Mental illness
- Blogs, vlogs and podcasts

Online Communities and forums:
- Side by Side (run by Mind)
- Big White Wall
- Beat message board
- SANE support forum

Medication

Another common type of treatment widely used is prescription medication. This can be used for various mental health problems with the ambition to lessen the effects of symptoms. Medication can't cure a mental health problem, but for some people they can help get you more stable. Medication helps with the biological component of the problem, but there needs to be a holistic approach, including reviewing your social circumstances and accessing psychological support. However, using medications makes the issue more manageable and can enable individuals to live happy, fulfilled lives. It is important to remember to take the medication that your doctor prescribes for you. Medication aims to ease the symptoms associated with poor mental health and assists in making life more manageable and enjoyable. For the best effects of any of these medications it is good to access self-help or psychological help to assist your journey.

There are a lot of misconceptions about medication so here are a few myths that need busting:

- Medication is a common form of therapy
- Does not make you a drug user
- It's not different than physical medication
- Taking medication does not mean that you are weak

Who can prescribe you medication?

- GP   • Psychiatrist   • Specialist Nurse Practitioner

Anti-depressants

Medication for depressive symptoms is called anti-depressants. It is thought that anti-depressants work via altering brain chemicals (neurotransmitters) which are closely linked to our moods and emotions. You may find that some types of antidepressant work better than others for your symptoms. It is like any form of help, you have to find your right fit!

Common anti-depressants are:
- Selective Serotonin reuptake inhibitors/SSRI's (common)
  e.g. Fluoxetine, Citalopram, Sertraline

- Serotonin-noradrenaline reuptake inhibitors/SNRI's (common)
  e.g. Duloxetine, Venlafaxine

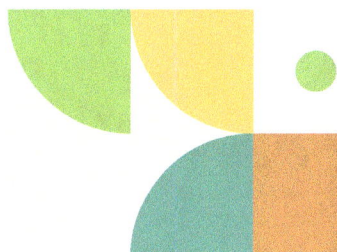

- Tricyclic anti-depressants/TCAs (less common)
  e.g. Amitriptyline

Anti-Anxiety medication

Like anti-depressants, these are aimed at reducing the symptoms of anxiety. They act through similar processes as anti-depressants. Often anti-depressant medication is prescribed for symptoms of anxiety because the symptoms are closely related. Often, anti-depressants are used for anxiety as there is some overlap in the receptors they target. Different medications are more helpful as anxiolytics (drugs used to reduce anxiety) – mirtazapine, venlafaxine or promethazine (an antihistamine). Duloxetine and sertraline are not commonly used for anxiety and are known to increase it in some patients. Here are a couple of the most common types:

- SSRIs (common)   e.g. Sertraline, Escitalopram, Paroxetine
- SNRIs (common)   e.g. Duloxetine, Venlafaxine
- Pregabalin (common is SSRIs and SNRIs are not suitable)
- Benzodiazepine (short term)

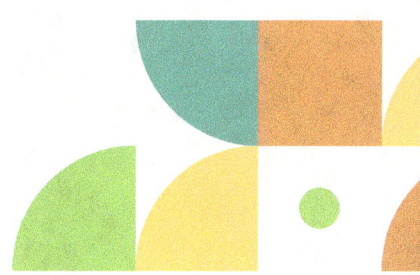

With all medication, it is important you do not self-diagnose or medicate yourself. You must go through trained medical professionals to help guide you in the right way and assist with any concerns you may have. It is also essential when you are prescribed any medication that you are in touch with your GP for assessment to monitor your overall wellbeing and progress. All medication comes with risk especially if you are already taking medication or have existing health concerns, you can always phone up your local pharmacist or GP for further assistance. Remember just because medication might have worked for someone else does not mean the same medication will have the same effect on you – everyone reacts differently to treatment and that is okay.

WHAT TO DO IN AN EMERGENCY?

In an emergency or crisis - you are completely warranted to call the emergency services. Here are some places you can go for support.

• Call 999 (Emergency Services) or go to Accident and Emergency

• Call the Samaritans on 116 123

• Text "SHOUT" to 85258

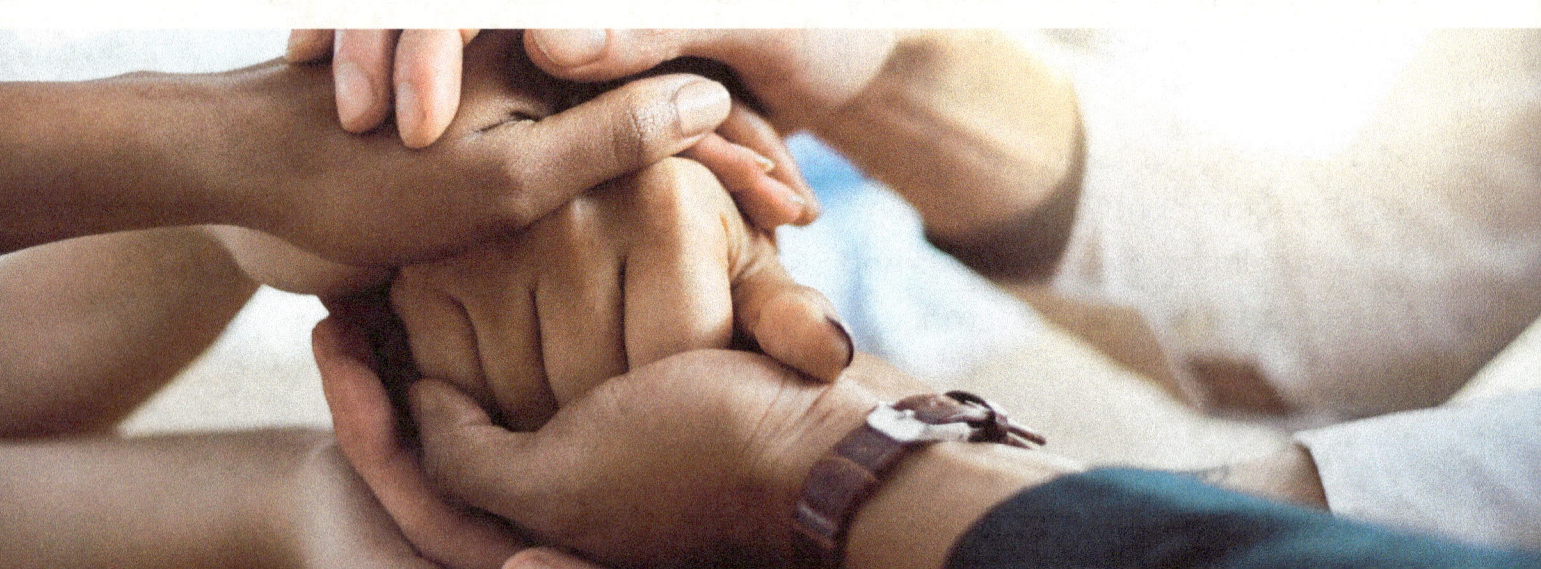

Building a Support Network

When you are going through a rough time it is important to have a support network around you to give you a hand if you need it. Support networks can be formal and informal and can come in a range of different settings. A good support system can look like anyone from a family member, a teacher or a colleague. They are those that you like, respect, trust and make you feel comfortable to talk to.

These are some benefits of a support network:

- Help with mental health and wellbeing
- Strengthen your immune system
- Lessening the effects of depression
- Lowering blood pressure
- Helping sleep problems
- Help with mood changes

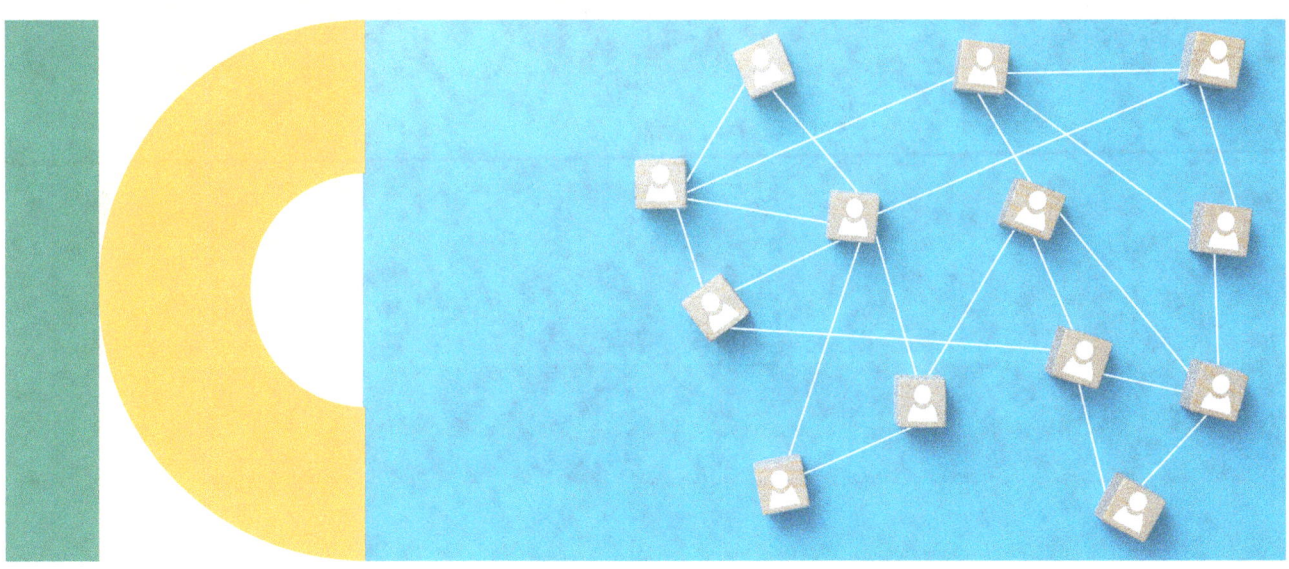

HERE ARE A FEW GOOD PLACES TO START WHEN MAKING YOUR SUPPORT NETWORK:

1. Reach out to family and friends
- They are people who care about you and want to know how to help.
- They can offer a helping hand without feeling judged.

2. Use technology
- Use messaging services to keep in contact with friends and family when you feel like you need to talk to them
- Online forums and chat spaces (check out the resources section at the back of the book).

3. Connect with people who share your interests:
- Volunteer groups
- Clubs and groups such as; dance, yoga and football
- Use a hobby to connect with others

4. Ask for help
- Places of worship
- Community centres
- Support groups
- Local mind shops and centres
- Libraries and community centres may have information for local services
- Your GP will be able to give you information about what is in your local area as well.

BUILDING A SUPPORT NETWORK

In the smaller boxes write in people whom you consider to be integral parts of your support network. In the larger box write all the positive benefits of having these support networks give you.

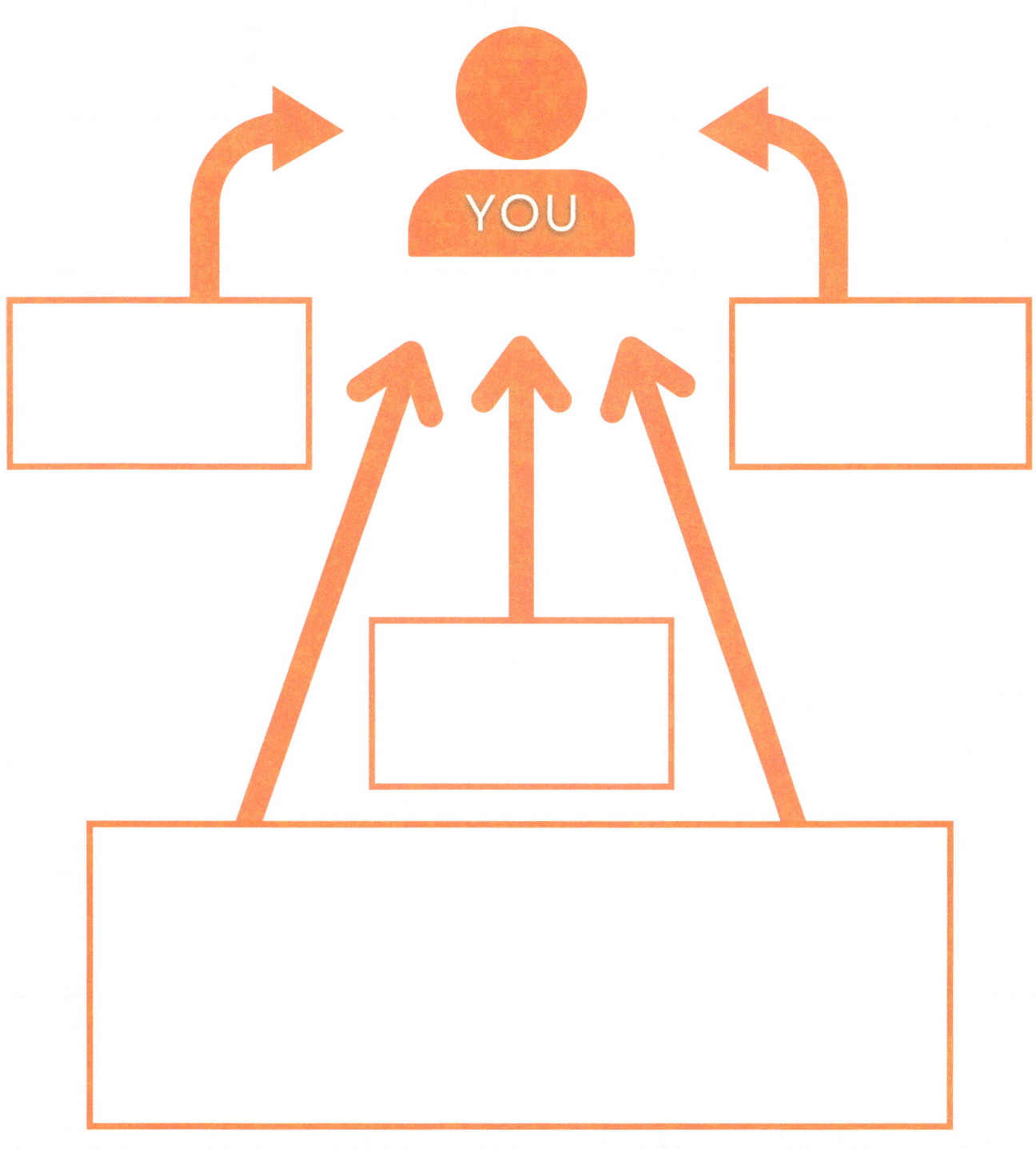

Creating and finding people for your support group might take some time. Remember to be kind to yourself and be patient. Just remember that everyone's support group looks different. It can be however big or small you like as long as it has people you trust. There are loads of people out there who are ready to help you; make sure you access them.

Visualising goals

Setting goals allows you to positively phrase the future and help your short-term motivation get there. It focuses your attention and resources, to get you where you want to go. Use these tips to help organize your time and monitor your process so that you can make as much progress as you can to your achievements. Remember it is okay to not achieve all the time. Life is not a linear path and sometimes a setback helps you phrase your actions in a different perspective. Remember to allow yourself to fail, to take time and to change directions. Try making a start with some SMART goals. To make each goal clear and reachable, each goal should be....

Specific
- simple, sensible and significant

Measurable
- meaningful, motivating and you're able to track progress

Achievable
- agreed upon, attainable and challenging but not too difficult based on your ability

Realistic
- reasonable, relevant, resourced, results-based. Think "is the goal actually possible for me to achieve?"

Time-bound
- time-based, time-limited and set a deadline

SPECIFIC:

....

MEASURABLE:

....

ACHIEVABLE:

....

REALISTIC:

....

TIME-BASED:

....

MY GOAL TRACKER

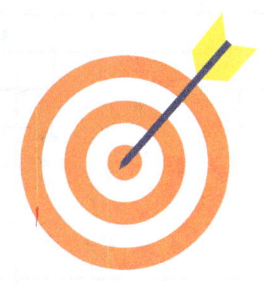

This month.....

I will do more

I will eat more

I will see more

I will try more

I will be more

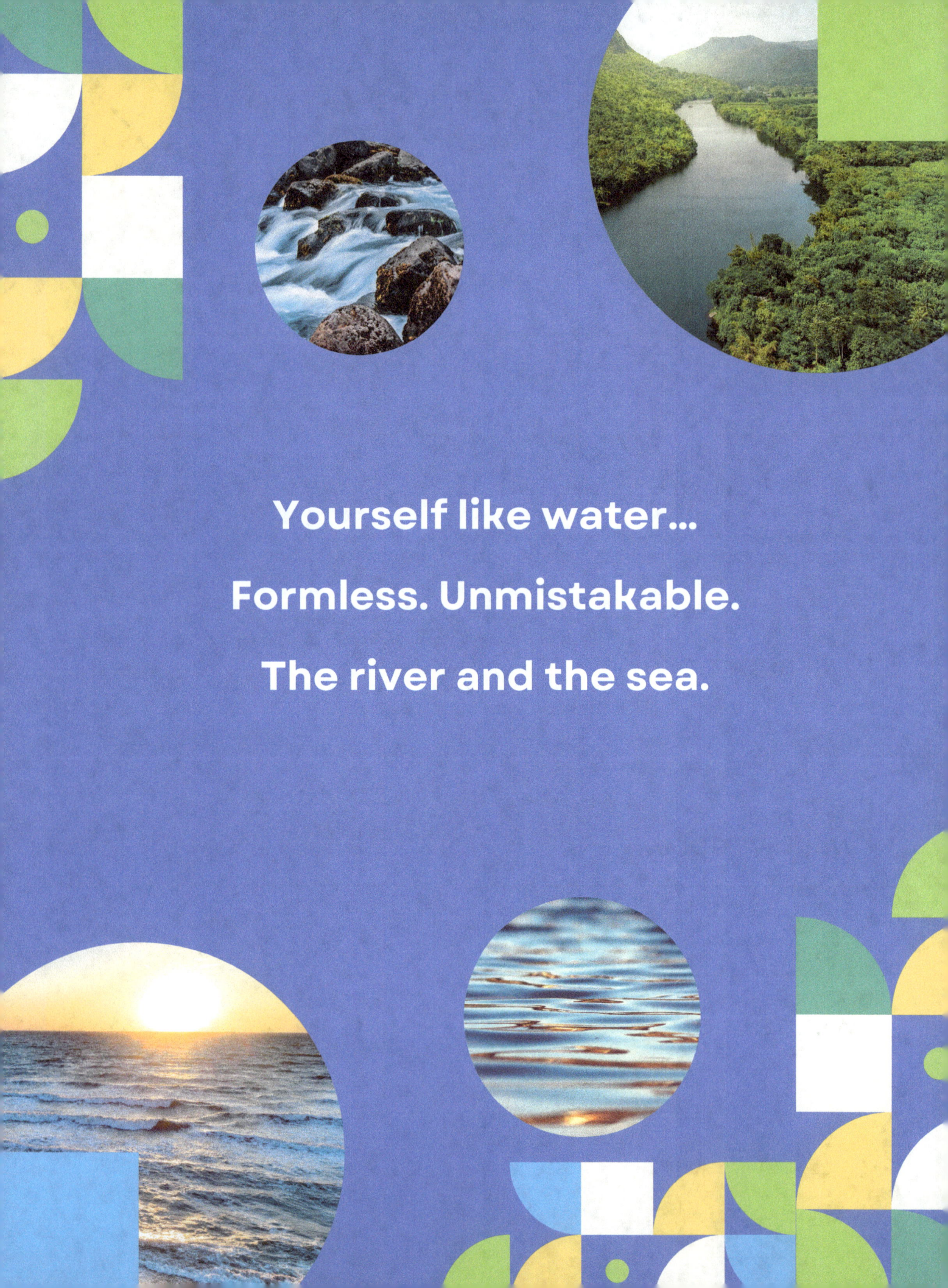

Yourself like water...

Formless. Unmistakable.

The river and the sea.

Acknowledgements

This incredible project would not have been possible without the help of many people. On behalf of Finn and I, we deeply thank the Be Free Campaign team for their overwhelming support in the production of this book. As part of the charity's passion for increasing access to mental health careers, we have partnered with Edge Hill University, where students come on board and complete a placement with us. Thank you to those students who have been involved.

Our clinical team have been phenomenal in giving advice and guidance on parts of the book. Our charity prides itself on evidence-based research and medical advice. Our clinical lead, Dr Kiron Griffin, psychiatrist Dr Shereen Hassan and nutritionist Nuna Kamhawi, have been wonderful in supporting and overseeing this project.

Our contributing authors have been inspirational and have been dedicated in their support of different sections of this book. This project could not have happened without the help of Zoe Edwards, Alizah Khan and Destiny Kumari who have shown overwhelming dedication to the production of this book.

Our editors have ensured that this book is digestible, informative, and engaging. Thanks to our editor in chief, Sarah Cornford, for her voice and guidance. Our editing team consisted of Aleena Siby, Zaynab Motala and Asheni Fernando - Thank you.

Our design team were monumental in coming up with a vision for this book - Katy Tudhope, Hanan Ajay and Morgan Morris.

Friends and family - thank you for all you have done in both our lives and the help you have given us in inspiring us to pursue our respective careers and develop our skills and passions.

Finally, thank you, to you the reader. Without your support, this would not have been possible.

MENTAL HEALTH RESPONDER

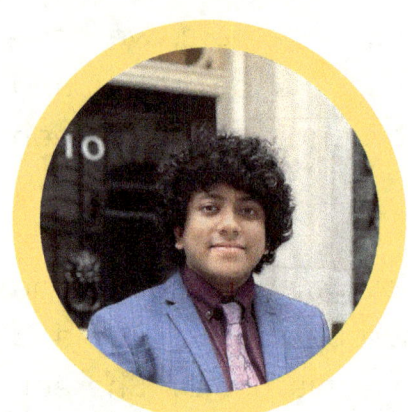

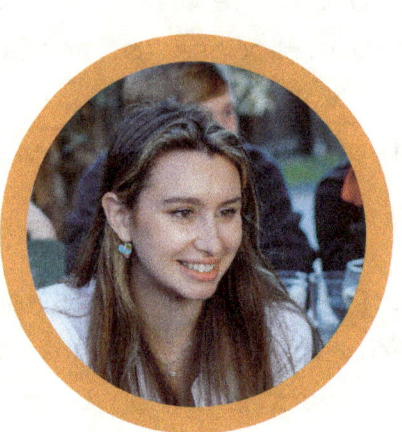

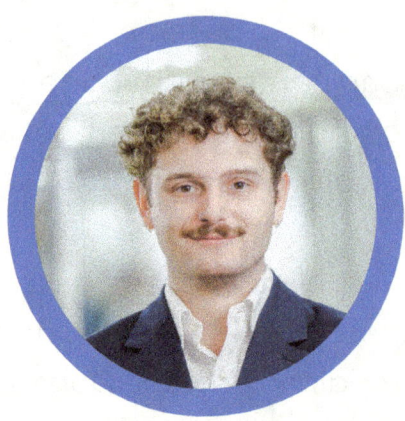

Shantanu Kundu
Chief Executive

Rachael Fell
Project Manager

Finn Thompson
Director of Strategy

RESEARCHERS & COURSE CREATORS

Dr Kiron Griffin   Lucy Tipple   Jaime Campfield

Soundarya Kandarpa   Emma Campbell   Holly Ennis

Louisa Clarke   Robert Chan   Holly Wilson   Yumi Livi

Haruko Cannon
Graphic Design

CONTRIBUTING AUTHORS

Dr Kiron Griffin (Psychiatrist and Public Health Specialist)
- Clinical Lead / Be Free Campaign

Dr Shereen Hassan (Psychiatrist)

Nuna Kamhawi (Nutritionist - ANutr)

Zoe Edwards

Alizah Khan

Destiny Kumari

Minnah Deef

Kelly Chang

Eleanor Gill

Rachael Dowling

Katie Mckenzie

Jordan Yeates

Haruko Cannon
(Graphic Design)

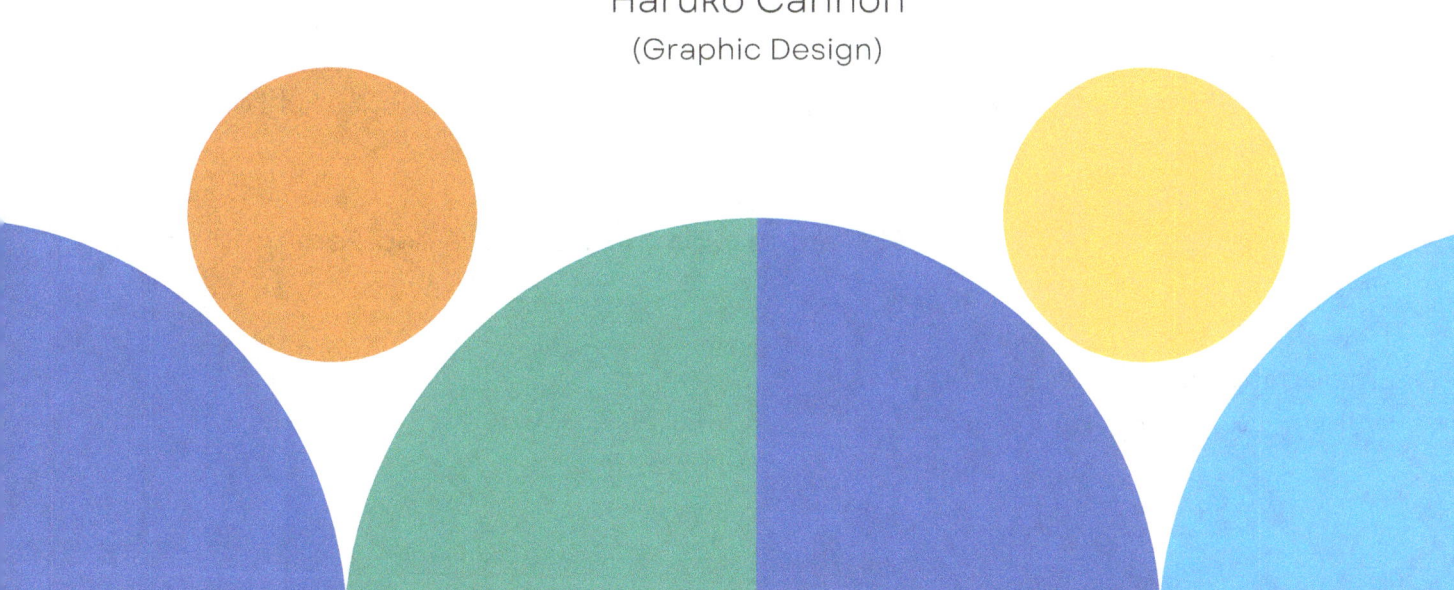

RESOURCES

Men's Health Forum

24/7 stress support for men by text, chat and email.
Website: www.mentalhealth.org.uk

Mental Health Foundation

Provides information and support for anyone with mental health problems or learning disabilities.
Website: www.mentalhealth.org.uk

No Panic

A charity that offers support for those suffering with panic attacks and obsessive-compulsive disorders (OCD).
Phone: 0844 967 4848 (daily, 10am to 10pm)
Website: www.nopanic.org.uk

OCD Action:

Supports those with OCD and provide information on treatment and online resources.
Phone: 0845 390 6232 (Monday to Friday, 9:30am to 5pm).
Website: www.ocdaction.org.uk

OCD UK

A charity run by people with OCD, for people with OCD. Provides facts, news and treatments.
Phone: 0333 212 7890 (Monday to Friday, 9am to 5pm)
Website: www.ocduk.org

Papyrus

The national charity dedicated to the prevention of young suicide. For children and young people under the age of
35 who are experiencing thoughts of suicide.
Phone: Help line UK 0800 068 4141 (9am to 10pm on weekdays and 2pm to 10pm on weekends)
Text: 07860039967
Email: pat@papyrus-uk.org
Website: www.papyrus-uk.org

Rethink Mental Illness

Offers support and advice for those who are living with mental distress.
Phone: 0300 5000 927 (Monday to Friday, 9:30am to 4pm)
Website: www.rethink.org

Mind

Promotes the views and needs of people with mental health problems.
Phone: 0300 123 3393 (Monday to Friday, 9am to 6pm)
Website: www.mind.org.uk

SANE

A national out-of-hours mental health helpline offering specialist emotional support, guidance and information to
anyone affected by mental illness, including family, friends and carers.
Phone: SANE line 0300 304 7000 (4:30pm to 10:30pm everyday)
Peer support forum: www.sane.org.uk/supportforum
Website: www.sane.org.uk

Support Line:

Provides a confidential telephone helpline offering emotional support to any individual on any issue.
Phone: 01708 765200
Website: www.supportline.org.uk

The Mix

For under 25.
Phone: 0808 808 4994 (Sunday to Friday 2pm to 11pm)
Website: www.themix.org.uk

Young Minds

If you are a young person experiencing a mental health crisis, you can text the Young Minds Crisis Messenger for free,
24/7 support. If you are experiencing a mental health crisis and need support.
Phone: Parents Helpline 0808 802 5544 (Monday to Friday 9:30am to 4pm)
Text: YM to 85258.
Website: www.youngminds.org.uk

NSPCC

Helpline. If you're worried about a child, even if you're unsure, contact our professional counsellors for help, advice
and support.
Phone: 0808 800 5000
Email: help@nspcc.org.uk
Website: www.nspcc.org.uk

Childline

A free, private and confidential service where young people can talk about anything.
Phone: 0800 1111, provides online 1-2-1 counselling and send email
Website: www.childline.org.uk

Refuge:

Advice on dealing with domestic abuse.
Phone: 0808 2000 247 (24-hr helpline)
Website: www.refuge.org.uk

Alcoholics Anonymous

A free self-help group for getting sober.
Phone: 0800 917 7650 (24-hour helpline)
Website: www.alcoholics-anonymous.org.uk

Al-Anon

A free self-help "12 step" group for anyone whose life is or has been affected by someone else's drinking.
Phone: 0800 0086 811 (daily, 10am to 10pm)
Website: https://www.al-anonuk.org.uk/

BEAT

The UK's Eating Disorder Charity
www.beateatingdisorder.org.uk

REFERENCES

Introduction

www.befreecampaign.org

Centres for Disease Control and Prevention (CDC). Well-being concepts (https://www.cdc.gov/hrqol/wellbeing.htm). USA: CDC; 2018 [cited 2020 November 17].

Gallagher, M., Muldoon, O. T., & Pettigrew, J. (2015). An integrative review of social and occupational factors influencing health and wellbeing. Frontiers in psychology, 6, 1281.

Michaelson, J., Mahony, S., & Schifferes, J. (2012). Measuring wellbeing: A guide for practitioners. New Economics Foundation, London.

Stevenson, A. (Ed.). (2010). Oxford Dictionary of English. Oxford University Press, USA.

Physical day-to-day wellbeing

Biddle, S. J., & Mutrie, N. (2007). Psychology of physical activity: Determinants, well-being and interventions. Routledge.

Nash, M. (2014). Physical health and well-being in mental health nursing: Clinical skills for practice. McGraw-Hill Education (UK).

https://www.medicalnewstoday.com/articles/290814#:~:text=Drinking water also keeps the,can also reduce tooth decay.&text=Blood is more than 90,different parts of the body.&text=With dehydration%2C the skin can,skin disorders and premature wrinkling.

https://solaramentalhealth.com/can-drinking-enough-water-help-my-depression-and-anxiety/#:~:text=Water has been shown to,can create feelings of relaxation.

https://www.nhs.uk/news/food-and-diet/six-to-eight-glasses-of-water-still-best/

https://www.ncbi.nlm.nih.gov/pmc/articles/PMC5876785/#:~:text=Based on literature our findings,associated with decreased immune responses

https://www.generalandmedical.com/live-healthy/posts/2020/april/the-importance-of-routine-for-your-mental-health/

https://www.timecamp.com/blog/2018/11/daily-routine/

https://www.medicalnewstoday.com/articles/290814#:~:text=Drinking water also keeps the,can also reduce tooth decay.&text=Blood is more than 90,different parts of the body.&text=With dehydration%2C the skin can,skin disorders and premature wrinkling.

https://solaramentalhealth.com/can-drinking-enough-water-help-my-depression-and-anxiety/#:~:text=Water has been shown to,can create feelings of relaxation.

https://www.nhs.uk/news/food-and-diet/six-to-eight-glasses-of-water-still-best/

https://www.ncbi.nlm.nih.gov/pmc/articles/PMC5876785/#:~:text=Based on literature our findings,associated with decreased immune response.

National Health Service, (2018). A guide to yoga [online]. Retrieved from: https://www.nhs.uk/live-well/exercise/guide-to-yoga/ [Accessed 10th January 2021].

Mason, (2017). How yoga can support mental health. Mind Body Health. Retrieved from: https://www.chopra.com/articles/how-yoga-can-support-mental-health [Accessed 12th January 2021].

Parle, P, (2020). Yoga. Retrieved from: https://www.khyayoga.co.uk/ [Accessed 10th January 2021].

Downdog., (2020). Yoga. Retrieved from: https://www.downdogapp.com/ [Accessed 12th January 2021].

Mental day-to-day wellbeing

Bhugra, D., Bhui, K., Wong, S. Y. S., & Gilman, S. E. (Eds.). (2018). Oxford textbook of public mental health. Oxford University Press.

Gillam, T. (2018). Creativity, wellbeing and mental health practice. Springer International Publishing AG.

Cheng, S. T., Tsui, P. K., & Lam, J. H. (2015). Improving mental health in health care practitioners: Randomized controlled trial of a gratitude intervention. Journal of consulting and clinical psychology, 83(1), 177.

Carpenter, D. (2020). The science behind gratitude: how to practice gratitude. Retrieved from: https://www.happify.com/hd/the-science-behind-gratitude/ [accessed 18 January 2021].

Augustus, J., Bold, J., & Williams, B. (2019). An Introduction to Mental Health. SAGE.

Ullrich, P. M., & Lutgendorf, S. K. (2002). Journaling about stressful events: Effects of cognitive processing and emotional expression. Annals of Behavioural Medicine, 24(3), 244-250.

Purcell, M. (2006). The health benefits of journaling. Psych Central.

Neff, K. (2011). Self-compassion. Hachette UK.

https://www.mindful.org/meditation/mindfulness-getting-started/

https://www.mindful.org/walk-this-way/

Cooper, B. B. (2020, June 30). What is Meditation & How Does It Affects Our Brains? | Buffer. Buffer Resources. https://buffer.com/resources/how-meditation-affects-your-brain/

Headspace (subscription required for full access)

Corrigan, P. W., & Rao, D. (2012). On the self-stigma of mental illness: Stages, disclosure, and strategies for change. The Canadian Journal of Psychiatry, 57(8), 464-469.

Janssen, M., Heerkens, Y., Kuijer, W., Van Der Heijden, B., & Engels, J. (2018). Effects of Mindfulness-Based Stress Reduction on employees' mental health: A systematic review. PLOS ONE, 13(1), e0191332.

Jorm, A. F., & Kitchener, B. A. (2011). Noting a landmark achievement: mental health first aid training reaches 1% of Australian adults.

Rüsch, N., Brohan, E., Gabbidon, J., Thornicroft, G., & Clement, S. (2014). Stigma and disclosing one's mental illness to family and friends. Social Psychiatry and Psychiatric Epidemiology, 49(7), 1157-1160.

Mind UK. (2020, November 22). Seeking help for a mental health problem: How can I open up to my family and friends? [Guide]. https://www.mind.org.uk/information-support/guides-to-support-and-services/seeking-help-for-a-mental-health-problem/talking-to-friends-family/

Mind Tools. (2020, November 22). Disclosing to others [Guide]. https://www.mindtools.com/pages/article/self-disclosure

https://littlecoffeefox.com/ultimate-bullet-journal-cheat-sheet/

Here is a tutorial by Ryder Carroll, the creator of bullet journals himself, on 'How to Bullet Journal': https://youtu.be/fm15cmYU0IM

If you're artistic, you might like AmandaRachLee.

YouTube: https://www.youtube.com/user/amandarachlee Instagram: @amandarachlee

If you're more of a minimalist, have a look at Reflect with Raksha

YouTube: https://www.youtube.com/channel/UCeZf0wLSKmLCF3qefpjfrxg Instagram: @reflectwithraksha

If you don't like using colour but still want to decorate, check out Pacific Notion Instagram: @pacificnotation

https://littlecoffeefox.com/ultimate-bullet-journal-cheat-sheet/

Catch It app - NHS. (2018, April 4). NHS.UK. https://www.nhs.uk/apps-library/catch-it/

Not feeling too great and when you need a helping hand

Beck, J. S., & Beck, A. T. (1995). Cognitive therapy: Basics and beyond (No. Sirsi) i9780898628470). New York: Guilford press.

University Of Hull, (2020). Reflective writing: What is reflection? Why do it? Retrieved from: https://libguides.hull.ac.uk/reflectivewriting/reflection1a [Accessed 10th February 2021].

Scott., (2018). Rumination and self- reflection- Is your thinking over the limit? Retrieved from: http://mindboosts.com/rumination-and-self-reflection-is-your-thinking-over-the-limit/ [Accessed 9th February 2021].

Catch It app - NHS. (2018, April 4). NHS.UK. https://www.nhs.uk/apps-library/catch-it/

Penna, G. L. (2017a, October 30). Attacking Anxiety with Thought-Catching. Gina Della Penna, LMHC. https://ginadellapenna.com/attacking-anxiety-thought-catching/ Dan-Glauser, E. S., & Gross, J. J. (2015). The temporal dynamics of emotional acceptance: Experience, expression, and physiology. Biological Psychology, 108, 1-12.

Lindsay, E. K., & Creswell, J. D. (2017). Mechanisms of mindfulness training: Monitor and Acceptance Theory (MAT). Clinical Psychology Review, 51, 48-59.

Reed, R. G., Weihs, K. L., Sbarra, D. A., Breen, E. C., Irwin, M. R., & Butler, E. A. (2016). Emotional acceptance, inflammation, and sickness symptoms across the first two years following breast cancer diagnosis. Brain, behaviour, and immunity, 56, 165-174.

Mind, 2018. Benefits F&Q. [online] Available from: https://www.mind.org.uk/information-support/guides-to-support-and-services/benefits-faq/about-this-information/ [Accessed 23 Jan 2021]

https://www.mindtools.com/page6.html#:~:text=Setting goals gives you long,the most of your life.

Websites

https://www.mindtools.com/pages/article/smart-goals.html

MIND, 2018. Online mental health tools. [online] Available from: https://www.mind.org.uk/information-support/tips-for-everyday-living/online-mental-health/online-mental-health-tools/ [Accessed 11th January 2021].

NHS, 2018. Mental health charities and organisations. [online] Available from: https://www.nhs.uk/conditions/stress-anxiety-depression/mental-health-helplines/ [Accessed 11th January 2021].

Mind Side by Side: https://www.mind.org.uk/information-support/side-by-side-our-online-community/

Counselling directory: https://www.counselling-directory.org.uk/?gclid=Cj0KCQiAvbiBBhD-ARIsAGM48bzK6kIdycoPZC-qxmA6KWQKThg7IHDdTFIfs-Tsw8VvvBRK9x4be5caAjFMEALw_wcB

THE NATIONAL INSTITUTE OF MENTAL HEALTH, 2020. Taking control of your mental health:Tips for talking with your health -care provider. US: Government Printing Office. Available from:https://www.nimh.nih.gov/health/publications/tips-for-talking-with-your-health-care-provider/index.shtml [Accessed 12th January 2021].

National Health Service, (2018). Benefits of talking therapy. Retrieved from: https://www.nhs.uk/conditions/stress-anxiety-depression/benefits-of-talking-therapy/ [Accessed 10th January 2021].

LEACH, J., 2015. Improving mental health through social support: Building positive and empowering relationships. 1st ed. London: Jessica Kingsley Publishers

Shout, (2020). Get help. Retrieved from: https://giveusashout.org/get-help/ [Accessed 10th January 2021].

Tyrer, P. (2015). Improving mental health through social support: Building positive and empowering relationships by Jonathan Leach. Jessica Kingsley. 2014.

Samaritans, (2020). How we can help. Retrieved from: https://www.samaritans.org/ [Accessed 10th January 2021].

Doran, G. T. (1981). There's a SMART way to write management's goals and objectives. Management review, 70(11), 35-36.

Mental health training online and face to face. MHFA Portal. (2021). Retrieved 7 February 2021, from https://mhfaengland.org/.

NHS England, (2018). Antidepressants – overview. Retrieved from: https://www.nhs.uk/conditions/antidepressants/ [Accessed 11 January 2021].

Mind, (2016). Psychiatric medication. Retrieved from: https://www.mind.org.uk/information-support/drugs-and-treatments/medication/about-medication/ [Accessed 11 January 2021].

SUPPORT SERVICES

BE FREE CAMPAIGN
www.befreecampaign.org

NHS
Life-threatening emergency

☎ 999

Urgent, non-emergency medical advice

☎ 111

Anxiety UK
www.anxiety.org.uk

A charity providing support to those who have been diagnosed with an anxiety condition.

☎ 03444 775 774

Monday to Friday = 9:30am to 10pm
Saturday to Sunday = 10am to 8pm

Samaritans
www.samaritans.org

Free 24/7 helpline for those feeling suicidal or in crisis

☎ 116 123

✉ jo @ samaritans

Bipolar UK
www.bipolaruk.org.uk

A charity helping people living with manic depression or bipolar disorder.

Shout
For anyone in crisis anytime, anywhere. It is a place to go if you are struggling to cope and you need immediate help.

85258
(24/7 crisis text line)

CALM Campaign

Webchat is Available

www.thecalmzone.net

Against Living Miserably, for those who identify as male in the UK who are down or have hit a wall for any reason.

☎ 0800 58 58 58

Daily= 5 p.m. to midnight

118

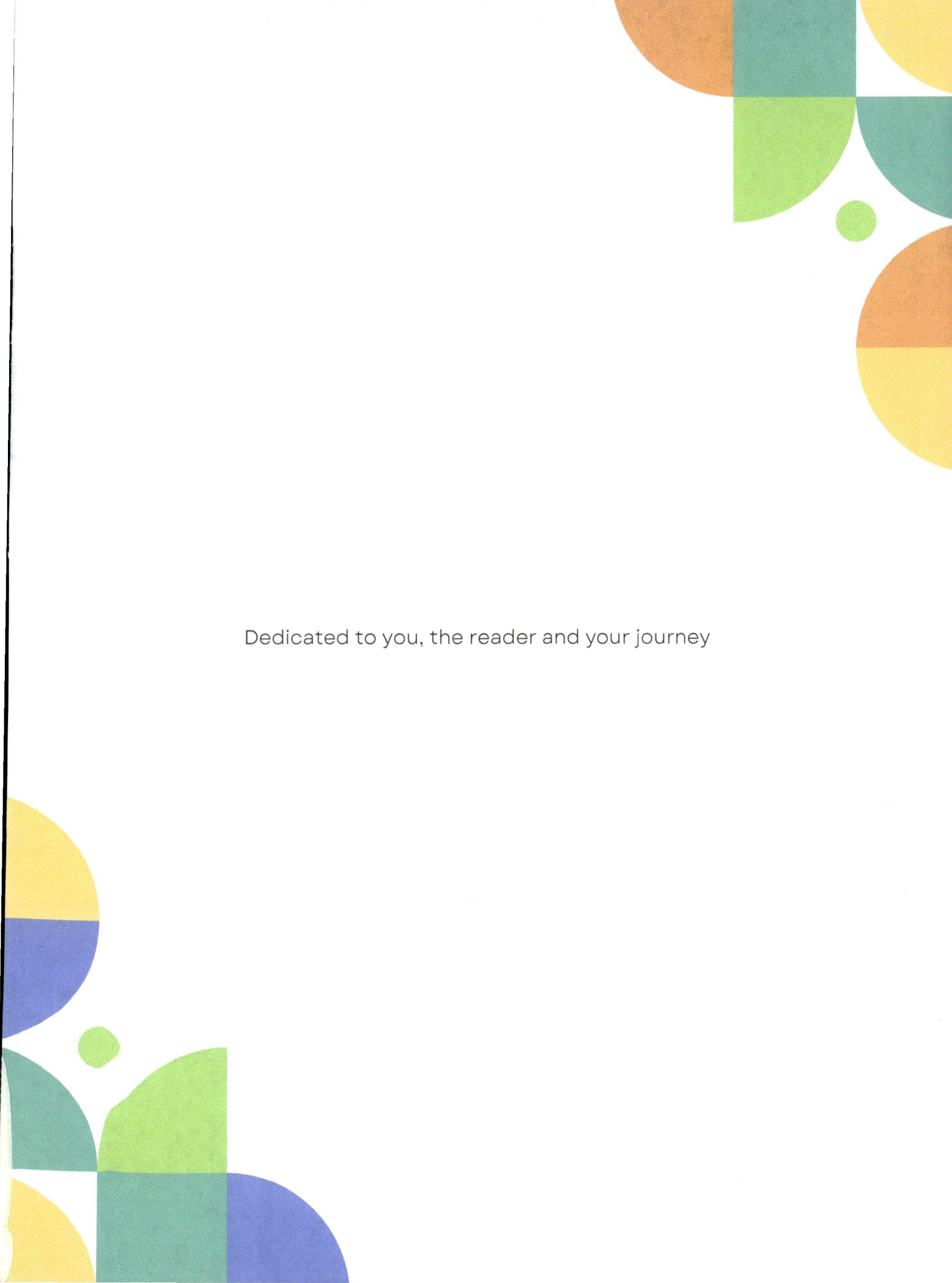

Dedicated to you, the reader and your journey